MY

BULLETPROOF

DIET

COOKBOOK:

(A BEGINNER'S GUIDE)

The Ultimate Guide to the Bulletproof Diet Recipes: Recipes to help you Lose up to 1LBS Every Day, Regain Energy and Live a Healthy Lifestyle.

By

Dave Scott

Disclaimer:

The information provided in this book is designed to provide helpful information on the subjects discussed. The publisher and author are not responsible for any specific health or allergy needs that may require medical supervision and are not liable for any damages or negative consequences from any treatment, action, application or preparation, to any person reading or following the information in this book.

Table of Contents

INTRODUCTION 7

> **STICK TO THE BULLETPROOF DIET TO KEEP LOSING A POUND A DAY, REGAIN ENERGY AND PUT AN END TO FOOD CRAVINGS** 7

BULLETPROOF DIET RECIPES YOUR DIET TO LOSING WEIGHT, UPGRADE YOUR LIFESTYLE AND END FOOD CRAVINGS FOR GOOD 10

> Avocado and Lump Crab Salad 10
>
> Zesty Lime Shrimp and Avocado Salad 11
>
> Summer Tomatoes, Roasted Corn, Crab and Avocado Salad 12
>
> Crab and Avocado Phyllo Bites 13
>
> Open Faced Tuna Sandwich with Avocado 14
>
> Zesty Avocado Cilantro Buttermilk Dressing 15
>
> Black Eyed Pea Dip 16
>
> Greek Nachos 17
>
> Guacamole Deviled Eggs 18
>
> Crock Pot Chicken and Black Bean Soup 19
>
> Cilantro Lime Tilapia Tacos 21
>
> Butternut Squash and Spinach Lasagna Rolls 23
>
> Tropical Fruit Salad Recipe 25
>
> Sautéed Julienned Summer Vegetables 26
>
> Slow Cooker Pork and Green Chile Stew 27
>
> Best Guacamole 29
>
> Shrimp Ceviche Cocktail 30
>
> California Grilled Chicken Avocado and Mango Salad 32
>
> Avocado Egg Salad 33
>
> Sugar-Free Chocolate Pecan Torte 34
>
> Peanut Butter Cups (Low Carb) 35
>
> Shrimp and Avocado Cocktail-tini Recipe 37

Holiday Vegetable and Hass Avocado Sauté Recipe 38

Mango, Papaya & Avocado Salsa Recipe 39

Meal in a Hass Avocado Half Recipe 40

Chilled Hass Avocado Soup Recipe 41

Cream of Avocado Soup Recipe 42

Gazpacho with Avocado Cream & Crispy Serrano Recipe 43

Quick and Creamy Avocado Soup Recipe 45

Avocado Spread Recipe 46

Avocado, Black Bean and Corn Salsa Recipe 47

Classic Guacamole Snack Recipe 48

Avocado and Cucumber Soup Recipe 49

Avocado and Tortilla Soup Recipe 50

Avocado Gazpacho with Peppadew and Coriander Croutons Recipe 51

Avocado Posole Recipe 53

Raspberry Avocado Salad with Honey Raspberry Vinaigrette Recipe 55

Roasted Beet and Hass Avocado Salad with Orange Dressing Recipe 56

Roasted Garlic Avocado Pasta Recipe 58

Tropical Salad with Hass Avocado and Grilled Shrimp Recipe 60

Hass Avocado Stuffed Marinated Mushrooms Recipe 62

Avocado and Turkey Crostini Recipe 63

Hass Avocado and Red Potato Salad Recipe 64

Raspberry Avocado Salad with Honey Raspberry Vinaigrette Recipe 65

Avocado and Tortilla Soup Recipe 66

Hass Avocado Board Guacamole Recipe 67

Antipasti Kabobs Recipe 68

Turkey and Avocado Sandwich Wedges Recipe 69

Meal in a Hass Avocado Half Recipe 70

Pork Fajitas with Hass Avocado, Red Onion and Tomato Recipe 71

Mama's Homemade Guacamole Recipe 73

Grilled Chicken Salad with Cranberries, Avocado, and Goat Cheese 74

Tomato, Turkey, And Avocado Open-Faced Sandwich 75

Spinach Salad with Avocado, Fresh Mozzarella, And Strawberry Dressing 76

Avocado with Black Bean Salad 77

Chicken, Mango, and Cheese Quesadillas 78

Key West Chicken-Avocado Sandwiches 79

Zesty Tofu, Avocado, and Quinoa Salad 80

Tomato Avocado Soup 81

Caesar dressing 82

Raspberry-walnut vinaigrette 83

Orange & Rosemary vinaigrette 84

Meat loaf with mushrooms recipe 85

Bean less chili recipe 87

Hearty beef stew recipe 89

Roast beef with thyme, garlic and red wine 90

Bacon-wrapped mini meatloaves Recipe 92

Sirloin Steak with Avocado Salad Recipe 93

Grilled Steak and Summer Veggies Recipe 94

Beef Brisket with Fall Vegetables Recipe 96

Bigos Recipe 98

Thai Pork Lettuce Wraps Recipe 99

Canned salmon salad 100

White wine & garlic mussels 101

Pork chops with apples and onions 102

Hearty beef stew recipe 103

Slow Cooker Beef and Pepper Soup Recipe 104

Steak with Bell Peppers Skillet Recipe 105

Texas-style of Beef Brisket Recipe 106

Gingered Beef Salad Recipe 107

Beef Chuck with Braised Vegetables Recipe 108

Bacon-Wrapped Butternut Squash Recipe 109

Spicy beef jerky 110

Thai Coconut Soup Recipe 111

Chunky Meat and Vegetable Soup Recipe 112

Creamy Zucchini and Mushroom Soup Recipe 113

Coconut Lime Chicken Soup Recipe 114

Bacon-Wrapped Avocado Recipe 115

Grilled peaches with Prosciutto and basil recipe 116

Avocado Daiquiri 117

Chilled Cucumber-Avocado Soup 118

Green Breakfast Burrito 119

Chocolate Avocado Shake 120

Tomato and Avocado Sashimi Salad 121

Egg, Avocado, and Spicy Mayo Sandwich 122

Carrot Soufflé 123

Cheesy Fried Rice 124

Chicken Nuggets fried in Coconut Oil 125

Chili-Coconut Crusted Shrimp 126

Chocolate Almond Granola 127

Roasted Red Kurri Coconut Curry Soup 128

Mango Coconut Chia Pudding 130

Better Bacon-Egg-and-Cheese Sandwich 131

CONCLUSION 132

INTRODUCTION

STICK TO THE BULLETPROOF DIET TO KEEP LOSING A POUND A DAY, REGAIN ENERGY AND PUT AN END TO FOOD CRAVINGS

Ask yourself the number of times you started out on a new diet with the greatest of intentions of getting healthier and losing weight only for everything to fall apart faster than you can say.

Dave Asprey in the bulletproof diet cookbook turned conventional diet wisdom on its head, outlining the plan responsible for his 100-pound weight loss, which he came to by "biohacking" his body and optimizing every aspect of his health. He urges for one to gain energy, build lean muscle, and watch the pounds melt off (just as he and so many of his devoted followers already have) you have to stop counting calories, eat high levels of healthy saturated fat, skip breakfast, work out less, sleep better, and add smart supplements.

The Bulletproof Diet could be called an "upgraded" Paleo diet. The condition is simple all you do is to eat a high (healthy!)-fat, low carb diet, getting **50-60% of calories from healthy fats, 20% from protein, and the remaining from vegetables**. A major disagreement between Bulletproof and Paleo is the ability to minimize toxins from the diet which are thought to play a major role in inflammation.

The bulletproof diet marked a significant moment in my approach to nutrition and health, and changed a lot of things in my life. You should understand that when it comes to losing weight, your diet is much more important than your exercise habits (for instance, losing weight is maybe 80% diet and 20% exercise). You can exercise all you want but if you're not taking care of your diet you are going to find it very difficult to strip off excess body fat.

The main reasons Paleo works well is because it removes grains from the diet, which are a very high source of mold contamination. Getting toxins out of your diet can effectively help you reduce inflammation and lose weight, even if you are not particularly sensitive.
This book is a great sit-down read, as well as a beginner's guide to the bulletproof diet.

This book contains other "hacks" as described in the Bulletproof Diet, which will make you feel really transform. I personally assure you that you will feel your best (sharper, happier, calmer) eating the high fat diet that Dave recommends in his book. I have recommended this type of diet to my clients and many have testified that the feel calmer, happier and have lost weight, without feeling hungry or unsatisfied.

However, if you have ever battled with weight issues, energy levels, focus throughout the day, mood swings, or any other nagging issues that you think might be holding you back, I highly recommend this book to you, and check out Even if you aren't actively working on

fixing one of those troubles, you owe it to yourself to try this stuff.
In addition, bulletproof Diet lets you experiment and change it up so that it works for you and your preferences. You do not have to count calories or measure your food. Instead, foods are arranged in a handy spectrum so you can choose in respect to how bulletproof you want to become.

To crown everything up, the diet recommends 60% of your diet should be "healthy" fat, 20% good quality meat, and the rest vegetables and a tiny bit of starch and It also promotes taking supplements. Have it in mind that there is No calorie counting, eat when hungry and stop when you're full and also No snacking between meals, and kick off the day with a bulletproof coffee.

BULLETPROOF DIET RECIPES YOUR DIET TO LOSING WEIGHT, UPGRADE YOUR LIFESTYLE AND END FOOD CRAVINGS FOR GOOD

Avocado and Lump Crab Salad

Ingredients:

About 4 oz. lump crab meat

1 ½ tablespoons of fresh lime juice (from a lime)

2 grape tomatoes (diced)

2 leaves butter lettuce (It is optional)

One medium Hass avocado (about 5 oz. avocado)

2 tablespoons of red onion (chopped)

1 tablespoon of fresh cilantro (chopped)

½ teaspoon of olive oil

¼ teaspoon of salt and fresh black pepper

Directions:

1. First, in a medium bowl, combine onion, cilantro, tomato, lime juice, olive oil, 1/8 teaspoon of salt and fresh pepper, to taste.
2. After which you add crab meat and gently toss.
3. After that you cut the avocado open, remove pit and peel the skin or spoon the avocado out.
4. Then you season with remaining 1/8 teaspoon of salt and fill the avocado halves equally with crab salad.
5. This makes about 2 servings, make sure you place on two plates with lettuce if you wish and serve.

Zesty Lime Shrimp and Avocado Salad

Ingredients:

2 limes (juice of)

¼ teaspoon of kosher salt (black pepper to taste)

1 medium tomato (diced)

1 tablespoon of cilantro (chopped)

¼ cup of red onion (chopped)

1 teaspoon of olive oil

1 lb. of jumbo cooked (peeled shrimp, chopped)

One medium hass avocado, diced (about 5 oz.)

1 jalapeno, seeds removed (diced fine)

Directions:

1. First, in a small bowl combine red onion, lime juice, olive oil, salt and pepper.
2. After which you let them marinate at least 5 minutes to mellow the flavor of the onion.
3. After that, in a large bowl combine chopped shrimp, jalapeño, avocado, tomato.
4. Then you combine all the ingredients together, add cilantro and gently toss.
5. Finally, you adjust salt and pepper to taste.

Summer Tomatoes, Roasted Corn, Crab and Avocado Salad

Ingredients:

1 pint grape tomatoes (cut in half)

2 hot peppers such as serrano or better still jalapeños, diced fine (seeds removed for mild)

1/3 cup of red onion (chopped)

1 teaspoon of olive oil

Salt and fresh pepper (to taste)

12 oz. lump crab meat

One hass avocado (diced)

1 ½ cups of roasted corn kernels

2 limes, juice of (or better still more to taste)

2 tablespoons of cilantro (chopped)

Directions:

1. First, in a small bowl combine red onion, olive oil, lime juice, pinch of salt and pepper.
2. After which you let them marinate at least 5 minutes to mellow the flavor of the onion.
3. Then in a large bowl combine chopped crab meat, avocado, tomatoes, hot pepper and corn.
4. After that, you combine all the ingredients together, add cilantro and gently toss.
5. Finally, you adjust lime juice, salt and pepper to taste.

Crab and Avocado Phyllo Bites

Ingredients:

¼ cup of minced red bell pepper

1 clove garlic (minced)

¼ teaspoon of kosher salt

½ medium (about 2 oz.) haas avocado, diced small

½ teaspoon of canola oil

¼ cup of onions (minced)

6 ½ oz. lump crab meat

1/8 teaspoon of black pepper

About 15 mini phyllo shells

Directions:

1. Meanwhile, you heat the oven to 350 degrees F.
2. After which you heat the oil in a sauté pan over medium heat.
3. After that, you sauté the onion, bell pepper, and garlic until soft.
4. Then you add the crab meat, salt, and pepper, and cook for about 30 to 60 seconds until the crab has been heated through.
5. At this point, you add about 1 heaping tablespoon of the crab filling to each phyllo shell.
6. This is when you arrange the stuffed shells on a baking tray, and bake for about 10 minutes.
7. Finally, you top each stuffed shell with avocado, and serve immediately.

Open Faced Tuna Sandwich with Avocado

Ingredients:

¼ cup of carrots (minced)

1 tablespoon of red onion (minced)

1 teaspoon of red wine vinegar

3 slices of multi-grain bread (toasted)

3 romaine lettuce leaves

0.5 oz. of alfalfa sprouts

5 oz. can albacore tuna (in water), drained

¼ cup of celery (minced)

1 teaspoon of Hellman's Light mayonnaise (or better still Greek yogurt)

Salt and pepper (to taste)

6 thin slices tomato

½ medium haas avocado (thinly sliced)

Directions:

1. First, you combine tuna with minced carrots, mayonnaise, celery, red onion, vinegar, salt and pepper.
2. After which you place lettuce on toasted bread.
3. Then you top with tomato, tuna, avocado and alfalfa sprouts.

Zesty Avocado Cilantro Buttermilk Dressing

Ingredients:

1 small jalapeno, seeds removed (feel free to leave them in if you want it spicy)

One medium haas avocado

2 tablespoons of scallion (chopped)

1/8 teaspoon of cumin

½ teaspoon of kosher salt

3/4 cup of low-fat buttermilk

¼ cup of fresh cilantro

1 clove of garlic

Juice of one lime

¼ teaspoon of fresh ground pepper

Directions:

1. First, you combine all the ingredients in a blender and blend until smooth.
2. However, if you want a thinner dressing, I will suggest you add more buttermilk, for a thicker dip use less.
3. It makes about 1-1/3 cups.

Black Eyed Pea Dip

Ingredients:

2 cloves garlic (crushed or minced)

1 Tablespoons of extra virgin olive

Pinch crushed red pepper flakes

1 cup of cooked corn, fresh or better still frozen, thawed

¼ cup of minced red onion (finely diced)

1 medium avocado (diced)

About 15 oz. of canned no salt black eye peas (Eden)

3 tablespoons of fresh lime juice (from about 1 ½ limes)

1 teaspoon of cumin

½ teaspoon of kosher salt

1 cup of cherry tomatoes (quartered)

¼ cup of cilantro (chopped)

1 jalapeño, seeded and better still diced (it is optional)

Directions:

1. First, you rinse and drain the black eyed peas in a colander.
2. After which in a large bowl, combine the garlic, oil, cumin, lime juice, crushed red pepper, and salt and mix well.
3. After that, you add the black-eyed peas, red onion, corn, tomato, jalapeno if using and cilantro.
4. Then you mix well and refrigerate at least 20 minutes.
5. Finally, when you ready to eat, gently mix in the avocado and serve right away.

Greek Nachos

Ingredients:

½ tomato (or better still ½ cup quartered grape tomatoes)

2 tablespoons of hummus (prepared or homemade)

Two small 100% whole wheat pita rounds (at about 70 - 80 calories each)

½ cucumber diced (at about ¾ cup)

¼ cup of crumbled feta cheese

Directions:

1. Meanwhile, you heat the oven to 375°F.
2. After which you cut the pita rounds into quarters and pull them apart so you have 8 triangles from each pita.
3. After that, you spread over a baking sheet and bake for about 8 to 10 minutes until toasted.
4. Then while toasting, combine the cucumbers, tomatoes and feta in a medium bowl.
5. Furthermore, you put the toasted pitas on two plates and drop some hummus onto the chips.
6. Finally, you spoon the tomato mixture on top and serve.

Guacamole Deviled Eggs

Ingredients:

One medium haas avocado

1 teaspoon of red onion (minced)

1 tablespoon of fresh cilantro (chopped)

Pinch Chile powder (for garnish)

6 large eggs (hard boiled)

2-3 teaspoons of fresh lime juice

1 tablespoon of minced jalapeno

Kosher salt and fresh ground pepper (to taste)

1 tablespoon of diced tomato

Directions:

1. First, you peel the cooled hard boiled eggs.
2. After which you cut the eggs in half horizontally, and set the yolks aside.
3. After that, in a bowl, mash the avocado and 2 whole egg yolks; discard the rest.
4. Then you mix in lime juice, cilantro, red onion, jalapeño, salt and pepper and adjust to taste.
5. At this point, you gently fold in tomato.
6. Furthermore, you scoop heaping spoonsful of the guacamole into the 12 halved eggs.
7. Finally, you sprinkle with a little Chile powder for color and arrange on a platter.

Crock Pot Chicken and Black Bean Soup

Ingredients:

3 ½ cups of low sodium chicken broth

1 red bell pepper (minced)

1 tablespoon of ground cumin

1 teaspoon of garlic powder

¼ teaspoon of oregano

½ cup of chopped cilantro (divided)

Cut limes (for serving)

Sour cream, for serving (it is optional)

2 (about 15 oz.) cans black beans (rinsed and drained)

2 (about 10 oz.) cans Rotel tomatoes with green chilies

4 oz. of can diced green chilies

1 teaspoon of ancho Chile powder

1 teaspoon of onion powder

About 16 oz. (2) skinless chicken breast

2 medium scallions (diced)

1 medium haas avocado (sliced)

Directions:

1. First, you take one can of beans and place in the blender along with 2 cups of the chicken broth; puree then add to your slow cooker.
2. After which you add the remainder of the beans and chicken broth into the slow cooker along with tomatoes, bell pepper, diced green Chile powder, chilies, oregano, chicken breast, cumin, garlic powder, onion powder, and ¼ cup of the cilantro.
3. After that, you set slow cooker to HIGH 4 hours or LOW 6 to 8 hours.
4. Then after it's done, you remove chicken and shred with 2 forks.

5. At this point, you place back into the slow cooker and add fresh scallions, remainder cilantro and adjust salt and cumin, to taste.
6. Make sure you serve hot with lime wedges, avocados, and sour cream if desired.
7. It makes about 10 ½ cups.

Cilantro Lime Tilapia Tacos

Ingredients:

1 teaspoon of olive oil

4 garlic cloves (finely minced)

2 cups of diced tomatoes

3 tablespoons of lime juice

8 5-inch of white corn tortillas (I prefer La Tortilla Factory Fiber and Flax)

Lime wedges and cilantro for garnish

1 lb. of tilapia fillets (rinsed and pat dried)

1 small onion (chopped)

2 jalapeño peppers, chopped (with seeds removed for less heat)

¼ cup of fresh cilantro (chopped)

Salt and pepper (to taste)

One medium haas avocado (sliced)

Directions:

1. First, you heat olive oil in a skillet.
2. After which you sauté onion until translucent, then add garlic and mix well.
3. After that, you place tilapia on the skillet and cook until the flesh starts to flake.
4. Then you add jalapeño peppers, tomatoes, cilantro and lime juice.
5. At this point, you sauté over medium-high heat for about 5 minutes, breaking up the fish with the spoon to get everything mixed well.
6. Furthermore, you season to taste with salt and pepper.
7. In the meantime, you heat tortillas on a skillet a few minutes on each side to warm (no oil needed).

8. Finally, you serve a little over ¼ cup of fish on each warmed tortillas with a slice or 2 of avocado and enjoy!

Butternut Squash and Spinach Lasagna Rolls

Ingredients:

<u>Ingredients For the Butternut Parmesan Sauce</u>:

1 teaspoon of olive oil

2 cloves garlic (minced)

Kosher salt and freshly ground black pepper (to taste)

1 lb. of butternut squash (peeled and diced)

¼ cup of shallots (minced)

2 tablespoons of fresh grated parmesan cheese

<u>Ingredients for the Lasagna:</u>

10 oz. package frozen chopped spinach (should be heated and squeezed well)

½ cup of fresh grated Parmesan cheese

Salt and fresh pepper

1 tablespoon of parsley (minced)

9 lasagna noodles, cooked (preferably use gluten free noodles for gluten free)

15 oz. of fat free ricotta cheese (I prefer Polly-o)

1 large egg

9 tablespoons (about 3 oz.) part skim shredded Italian Blend Cheese (I prefer Sargento)

Directions:

1. First, you bring a large pot of salted water to a boil.
2. After which you add butternut squash and cook until soft.

3. After that, you remove squash with a slotted spoon, reserve about 1 cup of the water and set aside, then blend until smooth with an immersion blender, adding ¼ cup of the reserved liquid to thin out.
4. In the meantime, in a large deep non-stick skillet, add the oil, sauté the shallots and garlic over medium-low heat at about 4 to 5 minutes until soft and golden.
5. Then you add pureed butternut squash, season with salt and fresh cracked pepper and add a little more of the reserved water to thin out to your liking.
6. Furthermore, you stir in 2 ½ tablespoons of the parmesan cheese and set aside.
7. Meanwhile, you heat oven to 350°F.
8. After which you ladle about ½ cup butternut sauce on the bottom of a 9 x 12 baking dish.
9. After that, you combine spinach, egg, ricotta, Parmesan, salt and pepper in a medium bowl.
10. At this point, you place a piece of wax paper on the counter and lay out lasagna noodles.
11. This is when you make sure noodles are dry.
12. In addition, you take 1/3 cup of ricotta mixture and spread evenly over noodle.
13. After that, you roll carefully and place seam side down onto the baking dish.
14. Make sure you repeat with remaining noodles.
15. Ladle about one cup of sauce over the noodles in the baking dish and top each one with 1 tablespoon of Italian cheese blend.
16. This is when you put foil over baking dish and bake for about 40 minutes, or until cheese melts and everything is hot and bubbly.
17. Finally, you top with parsley and serve (Makes about 9 rolls).
18. If you want to serve, ladle a little extra sauce on the plate and top with lasagna roll.

Tropical Fruit Salad Recipe

Ingredients:

Two mangoes, peeled and diced 3/4-inch cubes (about 2 ½ cups)

¼ cup of fresh grated coconut (for garnish)

One papaya, peeled and diced 3/4-inch cubes (about 5 cups)

One fresh pineapple, peeled and diced reserving the juice ¾ -inch cubes (about 4 cups)

Two large bananas, peeled and diced ¾ -inch cubes (about 2 cups)

Directions:

1. First, you combine the papaya, mangoes, and pineapple in a large bowl and add the juice from the pineapple.
2. After which you cover and refrigerate until chilled.
3. Then just before serving, I suggest you add the bananas and garnish with fresh coconut.

   Makes about 13 ½ cups.

Sautéed Julienned Summer Vegetables

Ingredients:

¼ cup of red onion (diced)

8 oz. of zucchini (cut into julienne strips with a mandolin)

Salt and fresh cracked pepper (to taste)

One tablespoons of extra virgin olive oil

3 cloves garlic (minced)

8 oz. yellow squash (cut into julienne strips, with a mandolin)

4 oz. (one medium) carrot, cut into julienne strips, with a mandolin.

Directions:

1. First, you heat a large nonstick skillet over medium heat.
2. Then when it is hot you add the oil, onions and garlic and cook about 1 to 2 minutes until fragrant.
3. After which you increase heat to medium-high and add the remaining vegetables, season with salt and pepper to taste and cook about 1 minute.
4. After that, you give it a stir to mix everything around and cook another 1 to 2 minutes, or until the vegetables are cooked through yet firm.
5. Finally, you adjust salt as needed and serve hot.

   Makes about 4 cups.

Slow Cooker Pork and Green Chile Stew

Ingredients:

Salt and pepper (to taste)

2 tablespoons of unbleached all-purpose flour

2 cans (about 4.25 oz. each) whole green chilies (sliced into thick rounds)

10 oz. can dice tomatoes and green chilies (Ro*Tel Mild)

1 tablespoon of cumin

Salt and fresh ground black pepper (to taste)

2 lbs. of boneless pork loin roast, lean, with all fat trimmed off

Cooking spray

¾ cup of diced onion

2 tablespoons of chopped jalapeño, or better still more to taste

½ cup of fat-free low-sodium chicken broth

½ teaspoon of garlic powder

Directions:

1. First, you cut pork into 2-inch pieces.
2. After which you season with salt and pepper.
3. After that, you heat a large non-stick skillet on high heat; when hot lightly spray the pan with oil and brown the pork over medium heat on all sides, about 3 - 4 minutes' total.
4. Then you sprinkle 1 tablespoon of flour over pork and stir to cook 30 seconds, sprinkle remaining flour over pork and cook an additional 30 seconds.
5. At this point, you add browned pork to the crock pot, along with the remaining ingredients.
6. Furthermore, you cook on LOW for 8 hours or HIGH for 4 hours (if you using a Dutch oven, I suggest you cook on low heat for about 3-4 hours).

7. Finally, when done, you adjust season, salt and pepper to taste if needed.

    it makes about 5 cups.

Best Guacamole

Ingredients:

1 lime (juiced)

1 small clove garlic (mashed)

Kosher salt and fresh pepper (to taste)

3 medium hass avocados (halved)

1/3 cup of red onion (minced)

1 tablespoon of cilantro (chopped)

Directions:

1. First, you place the pulp from the avocados in a medium bowl and slightly mash with a fork or a potato masher leaving some large chunks.
2. After which you add lime juice, cilantro, salt, pepper, red onion, garlic and mix thoroughly.
3. Then *if you are serving this at a later time, a great tip to keep the guacamole from turning brown is to cover tightly with plastic wrap so no air gets on it.*

    Makes about 2 cups.

Shrimp Ceviche Cocktail

Ingredients:

2 small limes (squeezed)

1 lb. large cooked shrimp (peeled and deveined)

One medium tomato (diced)

One serrano pepper (seeds removed and minced)

Salt and fresh black pepper to taste

2 ¼ cups of shredded iceberg lettuce

¼ cup of red onion (chopped)

1 teaspoon of olive oil

One medium hass avocado (diced into chunks)

One cup of diced English cucumber (not peeled)

2 tablespoons of chopped cilantro (plus more for garnish)

One lime cut into wedges for serving

Directions:

1. First, in a small bowl combine red onion, olive oil, lime juice, pinch of salt and pepper.
2. After which you let them marinate at least 5 minutes to mellow the flavor of the onion.
3. After that, in a large bowl combine shrimp, avocado, cucumber, tomato, Serrano pepper.
4. Then you combine all the ingredients together, add cilantro and gently toss.
5. At this point, you adjust salt and pepper to taste.
6. Furthermore, you fill nine martini glasses with shredded lettuce.
7. After that, you top each with ½ cup shrimp salad and garnish with a sprig of cilantro.

8. Finally you serve with a wedge of lime.

It makes about 4 ½ cups.

NOTE: make sure you weight after shrimp has been peeled.

California Grilled Chicken Avocado and Mango Salad

Ingredients:

1 cup of diced avocado

6 cups of baby red butter lettuce

12 oz. of grilled chicken breast, sliced (from 1 lb. raw)

1 cup of diced mango (from 1 ½ mangos)

2 tablespoons of diced red onion

Ingredients for the vinaigrette:

Salt and fresh cracked pepper to taste

2 tablespoons of olive oil

2 tablespoons of white balsamic vinegar

Directions:

1. First, you whisk vinaigrette ingredients and set aside.
2. After which you toss avocado, mango, chicken and red onion together.
3. After that, you fill a large salad platter with baby greens or divide on 4 small dishes; top with chicken/avocado mixture and drizzle half the dressing on top.
4. Finally, you serve with remaining dressing if desired.

Avocado Egg Salad

Ingredients:

4 hardboiled egg whites, chopped (make sure you discard the rest)

1 tablespoon of light mayonnaise

½ tablespoon of finely chopped chives

Pinch freshly ground pepper

4 large hard-boiled eggs (chopped)

1 medium hass avocado (cut into 1/2-inch pieces)

1 tablespoon of fat free plain yogurt

2 teaspoons of red wine vinegar

½ teaspoon of Kosher salt

Directions:

1. First, you combine the egg yolks with the avocado, chives, vinegar, light mayo, yogurt, salt and pepper.
2. After which you mash with a fork.
3. After that, you combine with egg whites and adjust salt as needed.

Sugar-Free Chocolate Pecan Torte

Ingredients

2/3 cup of cocoa

½ teaspoon of salt

1 cup (I stick) of butter, melted

½ cup of erythritol (it is optional)

1 cup of water

4 cups of pecans (make sure you don't use salted pecans!)

2 teaspoons of baking powder

8 eggs

2 teaspoons of vanilla

Artificial sweetener equivalent to 2 cups of sugar (I used zero-carb liquid sweeteners which was nice)

Directions:

1. First, you heat oven to a temperature of 350 F.

2. After which you grease an 8 or 9" round pan or spring form pan.

3. After that, you process pecans in food processor and then pulse until they are meal (note that they won't get quite as small as corn meal).

4. Then you add the rest of the dry ingredients and pulse again (note: I use more erythritol and is even better).

5. At this point, you add the wet ingredients and process until well-blended.

6. In addition, you pour into pan and bake. Remember, the exact time will vary with the pan and I suggest you start checking at about 25 minutes until toothpick inserted in center comes out clean.

7. Finally, you cut when cool and if you wish, serve with homemade whipped cream and/or chocolate sauce.

Peanut Butter Cups (Low Carb)

Notes:

1. However, these sugar-free, low-carb recipe cups are far better than any "diet candy" you can buy in a store.

2. In the other hand, you need a mini-muffin pan, preferably non-stick.

Ingredients

½ cup of heavy cream

Artificial sweetener equal to 2 cups of sugar (preferably, concentrated liquid Splenda)

2 teaspoons of vanilla

10 oz. of unsweetened chocolate

1 ¼ cups of powdered erythritol

½ teaspoons of salt

Ingredients for the filling:

2 cups of almond meal/flour

Dash of salt

1 cup of peanut butter

Artificial sweetener equal to 2 cups of sugar (preferably liquid sucralose)

Notes on the Methods and Ingredients:

It is essential not to overheat the chocolate, because chocolate melts at a little below body temperature. However, you don't need much heat. There are many ways you can melt chocolate, first, you can pour boiling water over it and then pour it off, you can heat the cream and then turn off the heat, or preferably use any method of your choice. Note that if you heat it too much it will separate and if this happens, I suggest you mix in a bunch of peanut butter and cut it into squares when cool. Or pour off the cocoa butter and put nuts in it along with the other ingredients for the chocolate outside, and it will be a very good fudge.

I recommend you use Hershey unsweetened chocolate because I figured it being readily available and if you use a higher-quality chocolate like Ghirardelli you will need more sweetener as much as half again as much of the zero-carb sweetener.

Directions:

1. First, you heat cream and the rest of ingredients and then turn off heat and add chocolate.

2. In the other hand, if you're melting it in the cream, I suggest you let stand until chocolate is melted -stir once in a while. Once it is all melted, mixture will be fairly thick. I will recommend you adjust sweetener to taste.

3. At this point, while the cream is heating and chocolate melting, I suggest you mix up the filling.

4. However, if it is too sticky, I suggest you put a little more almond flour or erythritol into it and then adjust sweetness (and possibly salt level) to taste.

5. After which you put heaping tablespoons or globs of the chocolate the size of a walnut into the mini muffin tin and then if it is thick enough you can sort of push out a place in the center and make the chocolate even around the sides. In addition, if it is not yet thick enough for this, don't worry, the peanut butter will push it up the sides.

6. After that, you form the peanut butter into smaller globs/balls and then push them into the chocolate, including pushing the top so it's flat.

7. Then you chill the whole thing in the refrigerator for half an hour or so.

8. This is when you remove from fridge and run hot water over the bottom of the pan for just a few seconds.

9. Finally, you take a thin knife and insert it at the edge of a cup.

10. Make sure you turn the whole thing a bit - then you know you can easily pop it out and if it doesn't work right away, I suggest you give it a few seconds so that the heat can penetrate, or it may need another shot of heat.

Shrimp and Avocado Cocktail-tini Recipe

Tips:

You can serve in martini glasses, this zesty shrimp and avocado cocktail is easy and elegant.

Ingredients

2 tablespoons of crushed garlic

½ cup of fresh cilantro, chopped (plus additional for garnish)

½ cup of ketchup

2 teaspoons of hot pepper sauce (or to taste)

4 ripe, Fresh Hass Avocados, plus additional for garnish

4 lbs. cooked shrimp (peeled and deveined)

2 cups of finely chopped red onion

3 cups of tomato and clam juice cocktail

½ cup of fresh lime juice

Salt and pepper to taste

Directions:

1. First, you place the shrimp in a large bowl.
2. After which you stir garlic, red onion, and cilantro.
3. After that, you mix in tomato and clam juice cocktail, ketchup, lime juice, and hot pepper sauce.
4. At this point, you season with salt and pepper.
5. Then you gently fold in avocado.
6. Furthermore, you cover, and refrigerate for 2 to 3 hours.
7. After that, you serve in martini glasses and garnish with cilantro leaves and more avocado slices if desired.
8. Finally, you serve with tostadas, corn chips, or crackers

Serving Suggestions:

Make sure you serve with tostadas, corn chips, or crackers.

Tips:

This recipe is colorful medley of zucchini, red bell pepper and Fresh Hass Avocado, perfect for holiday meals and year-round.

Ingredients

4 teaspoons finely chopped garlic

1 tablespoon of fresh thyme leaves

1 red bell pepper (cut into 1-inch squares)

2 ripe, Fresh Hass Avocado (seeded, peeled and cut into chunks)

3 tablespoons of avocado oil or olive oil

1 large shallot (finely chopped)

6 zucchinis (cut in half lengthwise and sliced 1/4-inch thick)

2 tablespoons of grated lemon peel

3 tablespoons of fresh lemon juice

Directions:

1. First, you heat oil in a large skillet over medium-high heat.
2. After which you add garlic, shallot and thyme, sauté for about 3 minutes.
3. After that, you mix in zucchini, bell pepper and lemon peel.
4. Then you stir and cook for about 2 minutes.
5. At this point, you lower heat and cover, cooking for about 3 minutes.
6. Furthermore, you combine in a small bowl the lemon juice with avocado.
7. Finally, you add to skillet and gently mix.
8. After which you cook for 2 minutes to allow flavors to blend.

Serving Suggestions:

Remember it will make a great accompaniment to roasted meat and poultry.

Mango, Papaya & Avocado Salsa Recipe

Tips:

This fruit salsa recipe calls for an extra burst of tropical fruit flavor from fresh papaya and avocado.

Make sure you serve in a dish for dipping or on your favorite grilled chicken or fish.

Prep Time: 10 minutes

Ingredients

2 ripe mangos (cut in ½- inch dice)

½ cup of diced sweet red peppers

2 tablespoons of minced jalapeño

2 lime (juice only)

2 ripe, Fresh Hass Avocado (seeded, peeled and cut in ½- inch dice)

2 ripe papayas (strawberry, if possible), cut in ½- inch dice

½ cup of diced yellow peppers

2 tablespoons of chopped cilantro

Directions:

1. First, you mix all ingredients and season to taste with salt and pepper.
2. After which you store in refrigerator until ready to use.

Tips:

This recipe will make an easy avocado vegetarian salad that is a meal in itself.

Remember that this avocado half filled with black beans and fresh salsa, this delightfully easy vegetarian meal can be enjoyed as a snack or as a fun first course at your next celebration.

Ingredients

1 cup of corn (drained)

½ cup of chopped fresh cilantro leaves

4 green onions (thinly sliced)

8 small bunches of radish or alfalfa sprouts

1 ¼ cups of black beans (rinsed and drained)

1 cup of packaged shredded carrots (lightly packed)

1 cup of prepared chunky salsa

20 drops of red pepper sauce

4 ripe, Fresh Hass Avocados (cut in half and seeded)

Directions:

1. First, you combine in a bowl the beans, cilantro, corn, carrots, salsa, green onion and red pepper sauce.
2. After which you fill each avocado shell with ½ of bean mixture.
3. Then you garnish with sprouts and serve.

Serving Suggestions:

Tip:

You should cut a thin lengthwise slice off of the bottom of each avocado half to make the avocados stable on the plates.

Chilled Hass Avocado Soup Recipe

Prep Time: 40 minutes

Ingredients

2 cucumbers (peeled, seeded and cubed)

4 cups of hand-torn romaine lettuce

4 scallions (thinly sliced)

2 cups of water

Lemon juice (to taste)

4 ripe, Fresh Hass Avocados (seeded, peeled and diced)

4 tablespoons of freshly chopped dill

2 medium green pepper (diced)

4 teaspoons of chopped garlic

2 fluid oz. vodka (optional)

Vinegar to taste

Directions:

1. First, you place all of the ingredients except vinegar and lemon juice in a blender.
2. After which you puree until smooth.
3. After that, you season with vinegar and lemon juice, to taste.
4. Note: the consistency of soup may be adjusted by adding more water.
5. Finally, you serve chilled.

Serving Suggestions:

Feel free to top with a spoonful of plain yogurt; garnish with chopped tomatoes and green peppers.

Cream of Avocado Soup Recipe

Tips:

This recipe can be pour into espresso or sake cups for a great addition to your party buffet.

Make sure you serve with mini breadsticks.

Ingredients

2 cups of cream

1 teaspoon of salt (or more to taste)

4 teaspoons of chives (chopped)

6 ripe, Fresh Hass Avocado (seed removed and peeled)

4 cups of chicken broth

4 tablespoons of fresh lime juice, or more to taste

Cream fraiche for garnish

Directions:

1. First, you place cream, avocado, chicken broth, salt and lime juice in a blender or food processor.
2. After which you blend until smooth.
3. After that, you taste and add more salt and lime juice if necessary.
4. Then you chill before serving with a tiny dollop of crème fraiche and a sprinkle of chopped chives.

Gazpacho with Avocado Cream & Crispy Serrano Recipe

Ingredients

4 (29 oz.) can fire roasted tomatoes

16 oz. of small red onion (diced)

2 stalk celery (diced)

Juice from 2 lime

4 tablespoons of sea salt

2 ripe, Fresh Hass Avocado (seeded and peeled)

6 tablespoons of goat cheese (soft)

6 slices of thin cut Serrano ham

2 (92 oz.) spicy vegetable juice

8 oz. small red bell pepper (diced)

24 oz. small hot house cucumber (diced)

6 tablespoons of fresh cilantro (chopped)

4 teaspoons of Black and red pepper blend

6 tablespoons of extra virgin olive oil

6 tablespoons of sour cream

2 tablespoons of lime juice

2 teaspoons of sea salt

Directions:

1. First, you combine in a large mixing bowl the vegetable juice, bell pepper, tomatoes, onions, cucumber, juice from 2 lime, celery, cilantro, cumin, Hot Shot, sea salt, EVOO and mix well.
2. After which you take out roughly 1/3 of the soup in food processor, or vita-mix blender, and pulse lightly on high for about 4-5 seconds until almost smooth.
3. After that, you add back to mixing bowl (Reserve for serving).
4. In addition, avocado cream- Cut in half, remove seed and flesh.

5. Then you place the flesh into a food processor with the sour cream, lime juice, goat cheese, and sea salt.
6. At this point, you puree until smooth (Reserve for serving).
7. Furthermore, crispy Serrano- in a large non-stick pan over medium heat, place sliced Serrano in pan and cook roughly 2 minutes per side until crispy (Note: make sure you cook like you would cook bacon).

If you want to serve-

1. First, you ladle soup into a chilled soup bowl.
2. After which you add a dollop of the avocado cream in the center and a piece of crispy Serrano ham on top of that.

Quick and Creamy Avocado Soup Recipe

Prep Time: 5 minutes

Total Time: 5 minutes

Ingredients

2 cups of vegetable or chicken broth (note: you should start by using 1/2 cup and add more per desired consistency)

2 tablespoons of non-fat plain Greek yogurt (or better still sour cream)

½ teaspoon of garlic powder

Salt to taste (preferably broth/bullion has salt, so may not be required)

2 ripe Fresh Hass Avocado (peeled and seeded)

2 teaspoons of lemon juice

1 teaspoon of herb of choice cilantro, basil, tarragon, dill (feel free to use more if fresh)

½ teaspoon of onion powder

½ teaspoon of Pepper

Directions:

1. First, you place all ingredients in blender and mix until smooth (note: you may garnish with avocado slices or cubes and dollop of yogurt or sour cream).
2. Make sure you serve warm or cool.
3. Remember that you may also use as a sauce for chicken, beef, fish or pork and is great on top of tacos!
4. I suggest you try this creamy soup or sauce as an alternative to traditional cream based soups and sauces!

Tips:

Remember that this fresh avocado spread recipe is a great addition to breakfast bagels or toast.

When you add to sandwiches and wraps for a creamy way to add naturally good fat.

Prep Time: 15 minutes

Total Time: 15 minutes

Ingredients

2 oz. Feta cheese

3 tablespoons of chopped chives or cilantro

Dashes of cayenne pepper

2 tablespoons of fresh squeezed lemon juice

2 ripe, Fresh Hass Avocado

½ teaspoon of onion powder

¼ teaspoon of black ground pepper

Sea salt to taste

Red pepper flakes (to taste)

Alternative Seasoning Options:

½ teaspoon of garlic powder in place of onion powder

½ teaspoon of lemon pepper in place of onion powder

Directions:

1. First, you combine avocado with goat cheese and mix until well blended.
2. After which you add remaining seasonings and mix well.
3. After that, you adjust sea salt and red pepper flakes to taste.
4. Then you garnish with fresh lime slices and a sprig of cilantro.

Avocado, Black Bean and Corn Salsa Recipe

Tips:

Remember that this colorful and versatile salsa is delicious any way you serve it (either as a dip, side dish, sandwich topper, or own its own with your favorite greens).

Prep Time: 15 minutes

Total Time: 15 minutes

Ingredients

½ cup of vinaigrette salad dressing

2 (about 30 oz.) can black beans (drained and rinsed)

Salt to taste

4 large (about 16 ounces) ripe Fresh Hass avocados (peeled and pitted)

½ cup of sliced scallions

2 cups of fresh or thawed and drained frozen corn kernels

1 cup of diced red pepper

Directions:

1. First, you cut avocados into 1/2 inch cubes.
2. After which you whisk together in large bowl the salad dressing and scallions.
3. After that, you stir in beans, corn and red pepper.
4. Then you add avocado; toss gently.
5. At this point, you season with salt, if desired.

NOTE: If you want to store, I suggest you place a piece of plastic wrap directly on the surface of the Salsa and refrigerate.

Classic Guacamole Snack Recipe

Prep Time: 10 minutes

Total Time: 10 minutes

Ingredients

2 teaspoons of lemon juice

40 (600g) baby carrots or approximately 8 large carrots cut into slices

2 ripe, Fresh Hass Avocado (peeled, pitted)

¼ teaspoon of garlic powder

¼ teaspoon of salt

Directions:

1. First, you mash in a large bowl the avocados with lemon juice.
2. After which you add in garlic powder and salt, mixing until combined.
3. Then you serve with carrot sticks, cherry tomatoes or your favorite fresh fruit or vegetable.

Serving Suggestions:

Remember, if the avocados were not refrigerated beforehand and you would prefer a colder guacamole, then I suggest you refrigerate the bowl of guacamole for about 15 minutes with a piece of clear plastic wrap pressed to the surface.

Note:

Remember that medium avocados are recommended for this recipe (medium avocado weighs about 5 ounces).

If you using smaller or larger sized avocados, I suggest you adjust the quantity accordingly.

Avocado and Cucumber Soup Recipe

Prep Time: 20 minutes

Total Time: 20 minutes, plus 1-hour chill time

Ingredients

2 cucumbers (de-seeded)

2 cups of plain Greek yogurt

2 whole wheat pita bread toasted

4 ripe, Fresh Hass Avocados

1 cup of Feta cheese

½ cup of fresh herb (basil, mint or cilantro)

Salt and pepper to taste

Note: If soup is too thick, I suggest you add 1 tablespoon of olive oil and pulse to combine.

Directions:

1. First, you peel and seed avocado then place avocado fruit in a food processor.
2. After which you add cucumber, feta cheese, yogurt and fresh herbs to food processor.
3. Then you blend until mix is smooth like a soup.

Serving Suggestions:

1. First, you adjust taste with salt and pepper.
2. After which you place in refrigerator for one hour before serving with toasted pita bread.

Avocado and Tortilla Soup Recipe

Prep Time: 20 minutes

Ingredients

4 cloves of roasted garlic

6 pt. of chicken broth

1 teaspoon of seasoned salt with red pepper frying oil

4 ripe, Fresh Hass Avocados (peeled, seeded and cubed or sliced)

4 limes (quartered)

1 cup of onion (minced)

2 tablespoons of olive oil

2 (31 oz.) can of tomatoes in juice (diced)

½ cup of coarsely chopped cilantro leaves

20 corn tortillas (day old) cut in strips

4 cups queso fresco cheese (crumbled)

Directions:

1. First, you sauté in a skillet, onion and garlic in oil for 1 to 2 minutes or until onion is transparent.
2. After which you place sautéed onion and garlic mixture with tomatoes in juice in a blender and blend for about 30 to 45 seconds.
3. After that, you combine in a stockpot the puree mixture, chicken broth, cilantro, and seasoned salt.
4. At this point, you bring to a boil, reduce heat and simmer for 10 minutes longer.
5. In the meantime, you heat 1-inch oil in a small saucepan.
6. Then when it is hot, you add tortilla strips a few at a time and fry, turn at least once; cook 1 to 2 minutes or until golden brown.
7. This is when you remove from oil with tongs and drain on paper towels.
8. Furthermore, you place equal portions of cooked tortilla strips in shallow soup bowls.
9. Finally, you ladle hot soup over, garnish with avocado, cheese and lime juice to taste.

Avocado Gazpacho with Peppadew and Coriander Croutons Recipe

Prep Time: 20 minutes

Ingredients

2 celery stalk

1 English cucumber

14 oz. apple juice

½ teaspoon of cayenne pepper

2 tablespoons of oil

4 green peppers (seeded and finely chopped)

8 ripe, Fresh Hass Avocados, mashed

4 tablespoons of fresh lemon juice

Salt and pepper to taste

Crouton Ingredients

10 peppadews

4 tablespoons of olive oil

Day old bread

Fresh coriander (to taste)

Directions:

First, you place all the gazpacho ingredients in a food processor and blend until smooth.

NOTE: if it is not a pouring consistency, I suggest you add a little water.

Then you chill in the refrigerator.

Crouton directions:

1. First, you cut day old bread into cubes, approximately 1-inch thick.
2. After which, you chop peppadews and fresh coriander to form a paste.
3. After that, you mix with olive oil.
4. At this point, you coat the cubes with the mixture.

5. Then you bake in the oven at 350 degrees F until crisp (note: make sure you toss the croutons regularly to avoid burning them).

Serving Suggestions:

You should pour the soup into chilled bowls and garnish with the croutons to serve.

Avocado Posole Recipe

Prep Time: 15 minutes

Cook Time: 20 minutes

Total Time: 35 minutes

Ingredients

2/3 cup of onion (diced)

2 jalapeño pepper

½ teaspoon of whole leaf oregano

½ teaspoon of ground white pepper

4 oz. canned green chilies (diced)

4 ½ cups of vegetable stock

6 tablespoons of fresh cilantro

2 fresh lime

4 teaspoons of olive oil

4 cloves garlic

1 teaspoon of ground cumin

2 ½ teaspoons of sea salt

½ teaspoon of cayenne pepper

12 oz. canned golden hominy (drained)

2 ripe tomato

4 Hass Avocados

Directions:

1. First, you dice the onions into ½ inch dice.
2. After which you mince the garlic.
3. After that, you stem and seed the jalapeno, finely minced.
4. At this point, you drain the green chilies and the hominy.

5. Then you chop the tomato and cilantro, set aside.
6. Furthermore, you cut the avocados in half and remove pit.
7. After that, you cut lime in half and rub the cut sides of avocado with the lime.
8. Mash 6 of the halves in a small bowl with the back of a fork.
9. This is when you cover surface with plastic wrap.
10. After that, you cover surface of remaining avocado half with plastic wrap.
11. Heat the olive oil in a 6 qtr. sauce pan over medium high heat until hot and add the onions, oregano, garlic, jalapeno, cumin, salt, white pepper and cayenne pepper.
12. Sauté for about 3 minutes until onion is soft.
13. Then you add the green chilies, hominy and the vegetable stock and bring up to a boil.
14. At this point, you reduce heat to a simmer and let simmer uncovered for about 15 minutes.
15. In addition, you remove from heat and add the mashed avocado, tomatoes and 4 tablespoons of the cilantro, stirring well to incorporate.
16. Finally, you juice the cut limes into soup.

Directions for serving-

First, you slice or chop remaining half of avocado and garnish top of soup with avocado and reserved cilantro.

Raspberry Avocado Salad with Honey Raspberry Vinaigrette Recipe

Ingredients

Salad

2 (10 oz.) package spring mix salad

1 cup of glazed walnuts (coarsely chopped)

Pepper to taste

4 ripe, Fresh Hass Avocados (peeled, seeded and diced)

2 (about 22 oz.) can mandarin oranges (well drained)

2/3 cups of sliced green onions

2 cups of fresh raspberries

Dressing

½ cup of raspberry vinegar

½ teaspoon of salt

½ cup of extra virgin olive oil

3 tablespoons of honey

1 tablespoon of Dijon mustard

Directions:

If you want to prepare dressing

1. First, you whisk together the oil, honey, vinegar, mustard and salt in a small bowl and set aside.
2. After which you place the greens, oranges, walnuts and onions in a large bowl.
3. After that, you drizzle with dressing and toss to coat.
4. Then you add avocados and raspberries and toss lightly.
5. Finally, you season to taste with freshly ground pepper.

Serving Suggestions:

Make sure you top with grilled chicken or salmon for a main meal salad.

Tips:

This recipe features a lovely mixture of avocados, rice vinegar, beets and orange zest sprinkled with homemade orange dressing.

This recipe is so tasty you wouldn't know it has only 120 calories per serving.

Prep Time: 10 minutes

Cook Time: 50 minutes

Total Time: 1 hour

Ingredients

Orange Dressing

4 teaspoons of white balsamic vinegar

¼ teaspoon of black pepper

½ cup of fresh orange juice

1 teaspoon of orange zest

½ teaspoon of salt

Salad

½ cup of seasoned rice vinegar

Orange zest (for garnish)

4 medium red beets

2 ripe, Fresh Hass Avocado (seeded, peeled and cut into quarters)

2 bag of mixed salad greens

Directions:

Directions on how to prepare dressing:

1. First, you combine in small bowl your orange juice, orange zest, vinegar, salt and pepper.
2. After which you whisk to blend and set aside.
3. After that, you wash beets and trim off stems.

4. Then you place beets in a small pan and add two tablespoons of water.
5. At this point, you cover pan with foil and roast in a temperature of 350 degrees F oven for 50 minutes.
6. After that, you check beets' doneness by piercing with fork.
7. At this stage fork should go in easily with a little resistance.
8. Furthermore, you remove from oven. Cool.
9. This is when you peel beets and cut into 1/4-inch chunks; set aside.
10. In addition, you dip avocado in rice vinegar and then divide greens among serving plates.
11. After which you top each serving with an avocado quarter and spoon 1/4 of the chopped beets over each avocado.
12. Finally, you drizzle dressing over all. Garnish with orange zest.

Serving Suggestions:

Tip:

If you want to make orange zest, use fine grater and grate off only orange color of skin.

Remember, there are also zest tools that you scrape on orange skin to make zest.

Roasted Garlic Avocado Pasta Recipe

Tips:

Remember that this pasta dish is chock full of flavorful fruits, chicken, vegetables and avocado.

Prep Time: 30 minutes

Cook Time: 15 minutes

Total Time: 45 minutes

Ingredients

2 Shallots thinly sliced (separated)

1 eggplant (cut in half lengthwise and sliced)

2 tablespoons of olive oil

16 oz. penne (or better still bow tie) pasta, cooked

1 lb. boneless, skinless chicken, cooked and cut into cubes

2 ripe Fresh Hass Avocado, seeded, peeled and cut into 32 slices

6 med. Zucchini (cut in half lengthwise and sliced)

2 med. red (or better still yellow bell pepper), cut into 1-inch pieces, membrane and seeds removed and thinly sliced

6 tablespoons of balsamic vinegar (divided)

10 cloves garlic (finely chopped)

1 lb. boneless, skinless chicken breast (cooked and cut into cubes)

1 cup of salt reduced, fat free chicken broth

Salt and pepper (to taste)

Fresh grated Parmesan cheese (to taste)

Optional chopped fresh basil or Italian parsley as garnish

Directions:

1. First, you bring a large pot of water to a boil over high heat.
2. After which you add pasta and cook according to package directions.
3. After that, you drain and cover to keep warm.
4. Then you sprayed in a large roasting pan with non-stick cooking spray, combine all vegetables.
5. At this point, you blend in a small bowl, about two thirds of the balsamic vinegar, oil, garlic, salt and pepper.
6. Furthermore, you pour over vegetables and toss to coat.
7. After that, you roast in preheated 375 degrees F. oven for about 45 min, stirring twice.
8. This is when you remove vegetables from oven and pour on remaining balsamic vinegar.
9. Then you toss together in a large bowl the cooked pasta, garlic and vegetables, chicken, and chicken broth
10. In addition, you portion into 16 pasta bowls.
11. Finally, you place two slices avocado and a fresh basil leaf on each.

Serving Suggestions:

Make sure you toss the pasta with fresh chopped basil for a different twist on the recipe.

Tropical Salad with Hass Avocado and Grilled Shrimp Recipe

Tips:

Remember that fresh tropical fruits topped with warm grilled shrimp make a perfect summertime salad.

Prep Time: 30 minutes

Cook Time: 5 minutes

Total Time: 35 minutes

Ingredients

Ginger dressing

4 mangoes, peeled, seeded and diced

2 ripe, Fresh Hass Avocado (seeded, peeled and cut into 1/4-inch slices)

2 lb. of medium or large shrimp (peeled and deveined)

1 pineapple (peeled, cored and diced)

2 papayas, peeled, seeded and diced

2 head butter lettuce (core removed, washed and chopped)

Ginger Dressing

6 tablespoons of finely chopped ginger

6 tablespoons of canola oil

4 cloves garlic

½ cup of coarsely chopped cilantro

4 lemons, zested and juiced

Directions:

1. First, you place shrimp a medium bowl.
2. After which you mix with half of the Ginger Dressing.
3. After that, you cover and refrigerate for about 20 minutes.
4. At this point, you thread shrimp onto pre-soaked wooden skewers.

5. Meanwhile, you heat a grill or grill pan to high heat.
6. Furthermore, you grill shrimp until cooked through, for about 2-3 minutes per side.
7. After which you remove from heat.
8. Then using a fork or tongs, I suggest you slide shrimp off of skewers and place shrimp in a bowl covered with foil to keep the shrimp warm.
9. After that, you toss together in a medium bowl pineapple, mango and papaya.
10. Then you divide lettuce equally among salad plates and top each plate with even amounts of pineapple mixture, avocado slices and shrimp.
11. Finally, you drizzle with reserved dressing.

Ginger Dressing

1. First, you place garlic, cilantro, ginger, lemon zest and juice, and oil in a food processor.
2. After which you blend until smooth.

Serving Suggestions:

Remember that the grilled shrimp can be served warm or cold with this salad.

Hass Avocado Stuffed Marinated Mushrooms Recipe

Prep Time: 20 minutes

Ingredients

1 1/3 cups of prepared balsamic dressing

2 teaspoons of coarse ground garlic salt

1 cup of crumbled feta cheese

4 (16 oz.) boxes fresh white mushrooms

2 tablespoons of fresh lemon juice

2 green onions (finely chopped)

4 ripe, Fresh Hass Avocados (halved, seeded and scooped out)

Directions:

1. First, use a wet paper towel to wipe all mushrooms to remove any soil.
2. After which you pop out mushroom stems.
3. After that, you place mushroom caps in a sealable plastic bag and add salad dressing, making sure all the mushrooms are coated with dressing.
4. Then you marinate the mushrooms for about 30 minutes.
5. This is when you remove mushrooms from dressing and set aside.
6. Furthermore, you combine in a medium bowl the lemon juice, garlic salt, onion and avocados.
7. After which you coarsely mash, combining all ingredients.
8. At this point, you spoon avocado mixture into a sealable plastic bag and seal tightly.
9. In addition, you push mixture away from one of the bottom corners of the bag.
10. Then with the help of a scissors cut a small hole in this corner of the plastic bag.
11. After that, you squeeze a generous amount of the avocado mixture through the hole in the bag into each mushroom cap and sprinkle with feta cheese.
12. Finally, you serve and enjoy.

Avocado and Turkey Crostini Recipe

Ingredients

Olive oil cooking spray

2 lemons (cut in half)

24 cherry or pear tomatoes (cut into small wedges)

2 French baguette

4 ripe, Fresh Hass Avocados

16 oz. sliced turkey (cut into 1-inch strips)

Directions:

1. Meanwhile, you heat oven to a temperature of 350 degrees F.
2. After which you use a serrated knife to cut baguette diagonally into thin slices.
3. After that, you lightly spray both sides with olive oil cooking spray and place on baking sheets.
4. Bake for about 8 minutes, or until light golden brown.
5. Then you remove from oven and let cool (NOTE: you can store these at room temperature in an airtight container for up to 2 days).
6. At this point, you cut each avocado into wedges and peel or cut off skin.
7. Furthermore, you cut into large pieces and squeeze lemon juice over avocado to prevent browning.
8. Finally, you place a strip of turkey on top of crostini and top with a few pieces of avocado and tomato.

Serving Suggestions:

1. Make sure you garnish this recipe with cilantro or flat leaf parsley if desired.
2. After which you use packaged crostini to make this easy hors d'oeuvre even easier.

Hass Avocado and Red Potato Salad Recipe

Tip:

Note that avocados add a tantalizing twist to traditional potato salad.

Prep Time: 15 minutes

Ingredients

2 cups of low-fat mayonnaise

4 teaspoons of Dijon-style mustard

1 ½ teaspoons of salt

4 ripe, Fresh Hass Avocados, seeded, peeled and chopped into 1/2-inch pieces

4 lbs. red potatoes (cut into 1-inch cubes)

10 teaspoons of cider vinegar

1 ½ teaspoons of ground black pepper

8 green onions (sliced)

Directions:

1. First, you place potatoes in a medium pan and cover with water.
2. After which you bring water to a boil and cook potatoes for about 15 minutes or until just tender when pierced with a fork.
3. After that, you drain well and pour into bowl.
4. At this point, you combine mayonnaise, mustard, vinegar, salt and pepper.
5. Then you add dressing and green onions to potatoes and gently toss.
6. This is when you stir in avocados.
7. Finally, you refrigerate for about 4 hours or overnight to allow flavors to blend.

Raspberry Avocado Salad with Honey Raspberry Vinaigrette Recipe

Ingredients

Salad

2 (10 oz.) package spring mix salad

1 cup of glazed walnuts (coarsely chopped)

Pepper to taste

4 ripe, Fresh Hass Avocados (peeled, seeded and diced)

2 (about 22 oz.) can mandarin oranges (well drained)

½ cup of sliced green onions

2 cups of fresh raspberries

Dressing

½ cup of extra virgin olive oil

½ cup of raspberry vinegar

3 tablespoons of honey

1 tablespoon of Dijon mustard

½ teaspoon of salt

Directions:

1. If you want to prepare the dressing, you start by whisking together the oil, honey, vinegar, mustard and salt in a small bowl; set aside.
2. After which you place the oranges, greens, walnuts and onions in a large bowl.
3. After that, you drizzle with dressing and toss to coat.
4. Then you add avocados and raspberries and toss lightly.
5. Finally, you season to taste with freshly ground pepper.

Serving Suggestions:

Make sure you top with grilled chicken or salmon for a main meal salad.

Avocado and Tortilla Soup Recipe

Prep Time: 20 minutes

Ingredients

6 cloves of roasted garlic

2 (31 oz.) can of tomatoes in juice (diced)

½ cup of coarsely chopped cilantro leaves

20 corn tortillas (day old) cut in strips

4 limes (quartered)

1 cup of onion (minced)

2 tablespoons of olive oil

6 pt. chicken broth

1 teaspoon of seasoned salt with red pepper frying oil

4 ripe, Fresh Hass Avocados (peeled, seeded and cubed or sliced)

4 cups of queso fresco cheese (crumbled)

Directions:

1. First, you sauté in a skillet the onion and garlic in oil for about 1 to 2 minutes or until onion is transparent.
2. After which you place sautéed onion and garlic mixture with tomatoes in juice in a blender and blend for about 30 to 45 seconds.
3. After that, you combine in a stockpot puree mixture, chicken broth, cilantro, and seasoned salt.
4. Then you bring to a boil, reduce heat and simmer for about 10 minutes longer.
5. In the meantime, you heat 1/2-inch oil in a small saucepan.
6. Furthermore, when hot, you add tortilla strips a few at a time and fry, turn at least once; cook for about 1 to 2 minutes or until golden brown.
7. At this point, you remove from oil with tongs. Drain on paper towels.
8. This is when you place equal portions of cooked tortilla strips in shallow soup bowls.
9. Finally, you ladle hot soup over, garnish with avocado, cheese and lime juice to taste.

Hass Avocado Board Guacamole Recipe

Prep Time: 10 minutes

Total Time: 10 minutes

Ingredients

2 tablespoons of fresh lemon juice

2 ripe Roma tomato (seeded, diced)

Salt and pepper (to taste)

8 ripe, Fresh Hass Avocados

1 small sweet white onion (minced)

4 serrano peppers (seeded if desired, diced)

½ cup of Cilantro, chopped, optional

Directions:

1. First, you peel, seed and gently mash all but one of the avocados with lemon juice in a bowl, leaving some chunks.
2. After which you gently stir in remaining ingredients.
3. After that, you peel, seed and dice remaining avocado.
4. Then you fold into the guacamole and serve immediately.

Serving Suggestions:

Make sure you serve this recipe with tortilla chips or add to your favorite meals - it's great with breakfast, lunch and dinner.

Antipasti Kabobs Recipe

Prep Time: 15 minutes

Total Time: 15 minutes

Ingredients

20 oz. salami

32 grape or cherry tomatoes

32 pitted Kalamata olives

Italian herbs (it is optional)

32 (about 6-in.) wooden skewers

4 firm-ripe, Fresh Hass Avocados (halved, seeded and peeled)

2 (about 8-oz.) package fresh mini mozzarella cheese balls

Olive oil spray or balsamic vinaigrette dressing mist

Directions:

1. First, you cut the salami into cubes or wedges about 1-inch wide (note: there should be enough for one cube per skewer).
2. After which you cut each avocado half into 24 chunks.
3. After that, you thread each skewer with a piece of avocado, followed by one grape tomato, a mozzarella cheese ball, another piece of avocado, one piece of salami, an olive, and a final piece of avocado.
4. Then you place skewers on a serving tray and mist lightly with the olive oil or balsamic vinaigrette dressing.
5. Finally, you sprinkle with chopped Italian herbs if desired, and serve.

Serving Suggestions:

It will be nice if you serve two kabobs crossed on a bed of greens for a pretty salad presentation.

Turkey and Avocado Sandwich Wedges Recipe

Tips:

Remember that these thick turkey avocado sandwich wedges are great for the lunch box or picnic basket.

Ingredients

2 ripe, Fresh Hass Avocados (peeled and seeded, divided)

3 (about 6 by 1 1/2-in) strips roasted red pepper

3 very thin slices red onion (halved and separated into rings)

2 romaine lettuce leaves

3 (about 1 ½ lb.) round flat sourdough bread loaves

3 Tablespoons of salsa

1 lb. of thinly sliced smoked turkey

3 (about 1-oz.) slices pepper jack cheese

Directions:

1. First, you cut a 4-inch circle out of the top of the bread; tear out the inside of the bread in the bottom section to make a shell.
2. After which you mash one avocado and mix with salsa; spread over the bottom of the bread.
3. After that, you layer pepper strips, onions, half the turkey, and then the cheese inside the bread.
4. Then you slice the remaining avocado and place on top of the cheese.
5. At this point, you top with lettuce and remaining turkey.
6. Furthermore, you replace the bread top and press down firmly to compress ingredients.
7. After that, you wrap tightly and refrigerate until ready to serve.
8. Finally, you cut into wedges just before serving.

Serving Suggestions:

Note:

Make sure you press the avocado mixture inside the roll to keep the air out, so these sandwiches can be made several hours in advance of serving.

Meal in a Hass Avocado Half Recipe

Ingredients

1 cup of corn (drained)

½ cup of chopped fresh cilantro leaves

4 green onions (thinly sliced)

8 small bunches of radish (or better still alfalfa sprouts)

1 1/3 cup of black beans (rinsed and drained)

1 cup of packaged shredded carrots (lightly packed)

1 cup of prepared chunky salsa

20 drops of red pepper sauce

4 ripe, Fresh Hass Avocados (cut in half and seeded)

Directions:

1. First, you combine beans, cilantro, corn, carrots, salsa, green onion and red pepper sauce in a bowl.
2. After which you fill each avocado shell with 1/4 of bean mixture.
3. Then you garnish with sprouts and serve.

Serving Suggestions:

Tip:

First, you cut a thin lengthwise slice off of the bottom of each avocado half to make the avocados stable on the plates.

Pork Fajitas with Hass Avocado, Red Onion and Tomato Recipe

Prep Time: 15 minutes

Cook Time: 5 minutes

Total Time: 20 minutes

Ingredients

2 oranges (juiced)

4 cloves garlic (crushed)

2 teaspoons of seasoned salt

2 tablespoons of canola oil

4 cups of cherry or grape tomatoes (sliced in half)

16 flour tortillas (warmed)

4 ripe, Fresh Hass Avocados (seeded and peeled)

2 lb. pork roast or tenderloin (trimmed of fat)

2 teaspoons of paprika

2 teaspoons of Pepper

2 small red onions (peeled and diced)

2 jalapeño pepper, seeded and minced (it is optional)

Directions:

1. First, you cut half the avocado into ½-inch cubes.
2. After which you place in a shallow bowl and pour orange juice over the avocado cubes.
3. After that, you slice remaining avocado; reserve.
4. Then you cut pork in strips about 1-inch by ½-inch.
5. At this point, you make in a small bowl a paste with the garlic, paprika, seasoned salt and pepper.
6. Furthermore, you rub paste all over pork strips.
7. After that, you heat oil in a large skillet over medium-high heat.
8. This is when you add pork and stir fry for two minutes, stirring frequently.

9. In addition, you add half of the diced onion and the jalapeño pepper to the skillet.
10. Then you cook and stir for two minutes.
11. After that you add half of the sliced tomatoes and cook for one more minute or until the pork is cooked through and the tomatoes are warm.
12. At this point, you gently stir in the diced avocado and juice.
13. Finally, you serve the fajitas with flour tortillas and garnish with the remaining onions, tomatoes and sliced avocado.

Serving Suggestions:

Make sure you serve this recipe with rice and vegetables for a zesty, easy-to-prepare meal.

Mama's Homemade Guacamole Recipe

Tips:

This recipe is a simple homemade guacamole, mild, easy and full of flavor.

Prep Time: 10 minutes

Total Time: 10 minutes

Ingredients

2 tablespoons of lemon juice

Salt and pepper (to taste)

8 ripe, Fresh Hass Avocados (seeded, peeled, cut in chunks)

1 small sweet white onion (minced)

2 ripe Roma tomato (seeded and diced)

Directions:

1. First, you mash avocados with lemon juice in a bowl, leaving some chunks.
2. After which you gently stir in remaining ingredients and serve immediately.

Serving Suggestions:

1. Remember that this mild guacamole can be customized easily to suit a variety of tastes.
2. First, you place small bowls of chopped jalapeño or serrano chilies, garlic, cilantro, tomato, onion, and seasonings around the guacamole bowl and let everyone build their own perfect dip.

Grilled Chicken Salad with Cranberries, Avocado, and Goat Cheese

Ingredients:

12 cups of arugula (1 prewashed bag)

1 avocado (pitted, peeled, and sliced)

¼ cup of walnuts (roughly chopped)

Salt and black pepper to taste

12 oz. of cooked chicken

¼ cup of dried cranberries

¼ cup of crumbled goat cheese

¼ cup of honey mustard vinaigrette

Directions:

First, you combine all ingredients in a large bowl, using your hands or two forks to fully incorporate the dressing.

Tomato, Turkey, And Avocado Open-Faced Sandwich

Ingredients:

4 tablespoons of hummus

2 tomatoes (sliced)

Salt and ground black pepper, to taste

4 slices whole-grain bread

1 avocado (sliced)

4 oz. of deli turkey

Directions:

1. First, you toast the bread.
2. After which you spread each piece with 2 tablespoons of hummus.
3. After that, you top with layers of avocado, turkey, and tomato slices.
4. Then you season with salt and pepper.
5. Enjoy!

Spinach Salad with Avocado, Fresh Mozzarella, And Strawberry Dressing

Ingredients:

2 Tablespoons of extra-virgin olive oil

1 Tablespoon and 1 teaspoon balsamic vinegar (divided)

1/ 8 teaspoon of freshly ground black pepper

1 ripe medium mango (peeled and cut in small chunks)

3 Tablespoons of chopped almonds (toasted)

2 chilled and sliced strawberries

2 Tablespoons of honey

½ teaspoon of salt

1 bag (6 ounces) of baby spinach

5 ounces of fresh mozzarella (cut in small chunks)

1 Hass avocado (peeled and cut in small chunks)

Directions:

1. First, you put ½ cup of strawberries, oil, honey, and balsamic vinegar in a food processor.
2. After which you process until smooth.
3. After that you scrape into a salad bowl and stir in the salt and pepper.
4. Then you add the spinach, mango, and remaining 1 ½ cups of strawberries to the dressing and toss to mix well.
5. Finally, you sprinkle the mozzarella, avocado, and almonds over the top.

Avocado with Black Bean Salad

Ingredients:

1 Tablespoon of lime juice

1 ½ Tablespoons of olive oil

1 can (15 ounces) of black beans (drained)

¼ green bell pepper (finely chopped)

1 garlic clove (minced)

½ teaspoon of salt

1/ 8 teaspoon of ground black pepper

1/ 8 teaspoon of ground red pepper (it is optional)

1 ½ teaspoons of chopped cilantro

1 avocado (quartered)

Directions:

1. First, you place the lime juice or vinegar in a large bowl and gradually whisk in the oil.
2. After which you stir in the beans, bell pepper, garlic, salt, black pepper, and red pepper.
3. After that, you taste and add more lime juice or vinegar if you like.
4. At this point, you stir in the cilantro.
5. Then you place the avocado, cavities up, on 4 plates.
6. Finally, you spoon the bean mixture into the cavities so it overflows onto the plate.

Chicken, Mango, and Cheese Quesadillas

Ingredients:

2 cups of shredded cooked chicken breast

2 tablespoons of chopped fresh cilantro

1 cup of shredded reduced-fat Cheddar cheese

4 multigrain wraps (10" diameter)

2 medium mango (sliced)

½ avocado (cut into 12 slices)

Directions:

1. First you arrange the wraps on a work surface.
2. After which you top the lower half of each wrap with ½ cup chicken, ½ cup mango, ½ Tablespoon cilantro, 3 slices avocado, and ¼ cup cheese.
3. After that, you fold the top half of each wrap over the filling to form a semicircle.
4. Than you heat a large nonstick skillet over medium heat.
5. In addition, you add the quesadillas and cook for about 4 minutes per side until lightly browned and the filling is hot.
6. Finally, you transfer to a cutting board, let stand 1 minute, then cut each into 4 wedges.

Key West Chicken-Avocado Sandwiches

Ingredients:

2 tablespoons of freshly squeezed lime juice

2 cup of baby spinach

8 small whole-grain rolls

2 cup of mashed Florida avocado (about 1 avocado)

1 teaspoon of green pepper sauce (it is optional)

20 oz. grilled or roasted chicken breast (sliced)

2 cups of mango (peeled, pitted, and sliced)

Directions:

1. First, you combine the avocado, lime juice, and green pepper sauce (it is optional) in a small bowl.
2. After which you spread the top and bottom halves of rolls with 2 tablespoons each of the avocado lime mixture.
3. After that, you layer ¼ cup of the spinach, one-quarter of the chicken, and ¼ cup of the mango on bottom halves.
4. Then you top with other halves of rolls.

Zesty Tofu, Avocado, and Quinoa Salad

Ingredients:

4 oz. extra-firm tofu (cubed)

6 tablespoons of diced green pepper

4 teaspoons of fresh lime juice

2 cups of cooked quinoa

6 tablespoons of diced red pepper

2 teaspoons of cilantro

4 tablespoons of diced avocado

Directions:

First, you combine all ingredients in a large bowl, toss to combine, and serve.

Tomato Avocado Soup

Ingredients:

1 sweet onion (sliced)

2 cups of water

2 cups of buttermilk

2 Hass avocados (sliced)

2 cans (about 28 ounces) of whole tomatoes

2 cups of reduced-sodium vegetable broth

1 teaspoons of ground pepper

½ cups of fat-free Greek-style yogurt

Directions:

1. Meanwhile, you heat the oven to a temperature of 350 ° F.
2. After which you pour the tomatoes (with juice) into an 11" x 17" baking dish.
3. After that, you scatter the onion on top and bake for 1 hour, or until the mixture is thick and the onion begins to brown.
4. At this point, you transfer the mixture to a blender.
5. Then you add the broth, water, and pepper and puree until smooth.
6. This is when you heat the soup mixture in a pot over medium-low heat for about 5 minutes, or until heated through and then add the buttermilk and stir to combine.
7. Finally, you garnish with each serving with 1 Tablespoon of the yogurt and ¼ of the avocado slices.

Caesar dressing

Ingredients

4 tablespoons of paleo mayonnaise

12 garlic cloves (minced)

Sea salt and freshly ground black pepper to taste

2 tablespoons of lemon juice

1 cup of extra-virgin olive oil

2 tablespoons of Dijon mustard Minced anchovy fillets

Directions:

1. First, with the use of a blender, process the lemon juice, garlic and mustard.
2. After which you add the paleo mayonnaise and blend again.
3. After that, you slowly add the olive oil while the blender is in motion.
4. At this point, you use a spatula to scrape all that delicious dressing in a bowl.
5. Then you season with salt and pepper.
6. Finally, you add some more lemon juice and some minced anchovy fillets to taste.

Raspberry-walnut vinaigrette

Tips: In this recipe the chopped walnuts give it a very nice texture.

Make sure you serve on a salad topped with extra walnuts.

Ingredients

1 teaspoons of Dijon mustard (it is optional)

Sea salt and freshly ground black pepper to taste

6 tablespoons of raspberry vinegar

4 tablespoons of chopped walnuts

1 ¼ cups of walnut oil

Directions:

First, you simply proceed in the same way you would for classic lemon juice vinaigrette and add the chopped walnuts at the end.

Orange & Rosemary vinaigrette

Ingredients

1 teaspoons of Dijon mustard (it is optional)

Grated zest and juice of 2 oranges

Sea salt and freshly ground black pepper to taste

6 tablespoons of fresh lime or lemon juice

1 ¼ cups of extra-virgin olive oil

2 teaspoons of chopped rosemary;

Directions:

1. First, you simply prepare classic lemon juice vinaigrette.
2. After which you add the grated zest and juice of one orange and 2 teaspoons of chopped rosemary. After that, you let infuse overnight for a better taste.

Meat loaf with mushrooms recipe

Ingredients
1 ½ teaspoons of sea salt
An egg
2 cups of white button mushrooms (finely chopped)
3 teaspoons of fresh thyme (minced)
3 cloves garlic (minced)
1 tablespoons of honey (it is optional)
1 tablespoons of paleo cooking fat
2 lbs. of ground beef (feel free to substitute with ground pork)
1 teaspoon of ground black pepper to taste
1 medium onion (finely chopped)
½ tablespoons of Worcestershire sauce (it is optional)
1 teaspoon of fresh oregano (minced)
½ cup of homemade ketchup
1 teaspoon of chili pepper flakes

Directions:
1. Meanwhile, you heat your oven to a temperature of 350 F.

2. After which you use a medium sized skillet placed over a medium heat, to melt the cooking fat, add the mushrooms and sauté for about 2 to 3 minutes, or until soft.

3. After that, you combine the meat, salt, pepper, egg, onion, mushrooms, chili pepper, thyme, oregano and garlic in a large bowl.

4. At this point, you mix well, making sure to break-up the meat.

5. Then you add the cooked mushrooms as well.

6. Make sure that the mushrooms are distributed evenly to ensure the loaf bonds well.

7. This is when you lightly grease loaf pan with additional cooking fat and fill it with the meat mixture.

8. After that, you place in the oven and cook for approximately 15 minutes.

9. Meanwhile, you combine ketchup, honey and Worcestershire sauce in a small bowl, to make the sauce for the top of the meatloaf.

10. After you might have cooked it for 15 minutes, you gently spread the sauce on the top of the loaf.

11. Then you continue cooking for another 40 minutes.

Bean less chili recipe

Ingredients
7 ½ lbs. of ground beef
9 cloves garlic (minced)
7 ½ celery stalks (chopped)
6 cups of button mushrooms (chopped)
4 ½ thyme sprigs
Sea salt and freshly ground black pepper to taste
4 ½ quarts good quality canned tomatoes
1 ½ tablespoons of extra-virgin olive oil
1 ½ onions (finely chopped)
7 ½ carrots (chopped)
4 ½ bay leaves
3 tablespoons of fresh parsley (chopped)

Directions:
1. First, you cook the ground beef with some cooking fat if needed in a large skillet over a medium heat.

2. After which you use a very large saucepan sauté the garlic in olive oil over a medium heat.

3. After that, you cook for about 2 minutes, or until the garlic is fragrant.

4. At this point, you add the onion, celery, carrots and mushrooms to the saucepan.

5. Then you stir well and cook for another 5 to 10 minutes, until the vegetables are soft.

6. This is when you add the canned tomatoes, followed by the cooked ground beef and then stir thoroughly.

7. Furthermore, you drop in the bay leaves, thyme and parsley.

8. After which you season to taste with salt and pepper, reduce the heat to low and simmer, uncovered, for approximately 4 hours or until thick, stirring occasionally.

9. After that, you adjust the seasoning by adding salt or pepper, if needed.

10. Finally, you remove the bay leaves and thyme sprigs.

Hearty beef stew recipe

Ingredients
4 tablespoons of paleo cooking fat
2 cups of onion (chopped)
6 carrots (peeled and chopped)
2 (28oz) can diced tomatoes
Sea salt and freshly ground black pepper to taste
2 lbs. of stewing beef
8 cups of beef stock
2 cups of celery (chopped)
4 potatoes, peeled and cubed (it is optional)
1 teaspoon of fresh rosemary (finely chopped)
1 teaspoon of fresh thyme (finely chopped)

Directions:
1. First, you combine the onions, celery, carrots, potatoes, if using, as well as the cooking fat in a large saucepan over a medium-high heat.

2. After which you cook for about 3 to 5 minutes, stirring constantly.

3. After that, you add the beef to the saucepan, followed by the tomatoes, beef stock, rosemary and thyme.

4. At this point, you season to taste with salt and pepper.

5. Then you cover the saucepan and cook for about one hour, allowing the stew to simmer.

6. This is when you stir a few times during the cooking process.

7. Finally, you remove the lid and cook uncovered for about 45 minutes and if the mixture is too thick at the end of the cooking process, I suggest you add a little bit of water or stock.

Roast beef with thyme, garlic and red wine

Ingredients
1 cup of clarified butter (or beef tallow)
6 cloves garlic (minced)
Sea salt and freshly ground black pepper to taste
2 (4lbs) top sirloin roast
6 tablespoons of homemade Worcestershire sauce (it is optional)
6 sprigs fresh thyme
1 ¼ cups of red wine

Directions:
1. Meanwhile, you heat your oven to a temperature of 350 F.

2. After which you melt 2 tablespoons of the cooking fat in a large skillet over high heat.

3. After that, you sear the roast on all sides for just a few moments, or until the sides are a beautiful golden brown.

4. Then you place the roast in a large roasting dish, along with the cooking fat used to sear it.

5. At this point, you scatter generous knobs of the cooking fat on top of the roast, followed by the Worcestershire sauce, if using, and red wine.

6. Furthermore, you sprinkle the garlic over the meat and season to taste with salt and pepper.

7. After which you top with the thyme sprigs.

8. After that, you allow to cook for about 50-60 minutes, or until the meat is cooked, but still slightly pink in the middle.

9. This is the point when you baste the meat with the cooking juices from time to time during the cooking process to ensure that the meat stays moist.

10. Then you remove the roast from the oven and set aside for about 10 minutes before serving, allowing the meat to relax before carving it.

11. Finally, you remove the thyme springs from the pan and use the rendered liquid in the pan as a sauce for the roast.

Bacon-wrapped mini meatloaves Recipe

Ingredients
1lb. of bacon (cut in small chunks)
½ cup of coconut milk
2/3 cup of fresh chives (minced)
Freshly ground black pepper to taste
2 lbs. of ground beef
16 additional strips of bacons
4 garlic cloves (minced)
Fresh parsley (chopped)

Directions:
1. Meanwhile, you heat your oven to a temperature of 400 F.

2. After which you combine the ground beef, the bacon chunks, the garlic, the chives and the coconut Milk in a big bowl.

3. After that, you mix well until all the ingredients hold together. To save yourself some time, I suggest you use an electric mixer.

4. At this point, you season the mixture with freshly ground black pepper to taste. Do not add salt to the mixture since the bacon is already salty enough.

5. Then you take a medium size muffin tin and place a slice of bacon around the sides of each hole.

6. Furthermore, you fill these same eight holes with the beef mixture.

7. After that, you place in the oven and cook for about 30 minutes.

8. Then once it is ready and cool enough to handle, you remove the mini meatloaves from the muffin tin and serve with fresh parsley sprinkled on top.

Sirloin Steak with Avocado Salad Recipe

Ingredients
2 avocados (peeled and diced)
1 cup of celery (sliced)
4 tablespoons of extra virgin olive oil
Sea salt and freshly ground black pepper to taste
4 big sirloin steaks
2 big red bell pepper (diced)
4 green onions (chopped)
2 tablespoons of lemon juice
4 tablespoons of Paleo cooking fat

Directions:
1. First, you use a skillet big enough to cook two steaks, melt 2 tablespoons of the cooking fat over medium-high heat.

2. After which you cook the red bell peppers for about 2 to 3 minutes until soft but still crunchy and set aside.

3. After that, you season the 4 steaks with sea salt and freshly ground black pepper to taste.

4. Then you use the same skillet, add the cooking fat and brown the two sirloins on each side, until done to your liking. Have in mind that in 2-3 minutes on each side will give you a nice medium-rare steak.

5. At this point, you remove the steaks from the skillet and let them rest for about 5 minutes.

6. This is when you combine the roasted red bell peppers, the green onions, the avocado, the celery, the lemon juice, and the olive oil, to prepare the salad in a big bowl.

7. After that, you season to taste with sea salt and freshly ground black pepper.

8. Finally, you cut the steak into slices, and serve with the avocado salad on top.

Grilled Steak and Summer Veggies Recipe

Ingredients
Four small zucchini (cut lengthwise)
2 cups of grape tomatoes (halved)
Fresh Herbs Vinaigrette
1 ½ lbs. of beef flank steak
½ cup of red onions (chopped)
4 big carrots (cut lengthwise)

Ingredients
½ cup of fresh basil (chopped)
1 teaspoons of Dijon mustard
Sea salt and freshly ground black pepper to taste
½ cup of fresh parsley (chopped)
1 clove garlic (chopped)
6 tablespoons of extra virgin olive oil
Juice from ½ a lemon

Directions:
1. First, you combine the entire ingredients for the vinaigrette except for the olive oil in a food processor.

2. After which you blend the entire ingredients for one minute, and then slowly pour in the olive oil.

3. At this point, you transfer to a bowl and reserve.

4. Meanwhile, you heat the grill to a medium-high heat.

5. After which you grill the flank steak for about 8 minutes for medium rare or more if you like it well done.

6. At a point, once it is cooked, you remove from the grill and set aside to rest.

7. After that, you combine the zucchini, the carrots, the red onions and 1 tablespoons of the vinaigrette and combine well.

8. Then you place the vegetables on the grill and cook for about 5 to 6 minutes, flipping them once.

9. Furthermore, you cut the cooked steak into slices and, in a big bowl, combine the steak, the cooked vegetables, and the grape tomatoes.

10. Finally, you add the remaining vinaigrette and toss to mix.

   10. After which you season to taste with sea salt and black pepper before serving.

Beef Brisket with Fall Vegetables Recipe

Ingredients
4 carrots (cut into 2-inch pieces)
2 celery ribs (sliced)
1 leek (sliced)
2 cups of beef stock (preferably, 3 cups if not using wine)
½ cups of tomato puree
8 garlic cloves (minced)
Sea Salt and freshly ground black pepper to taste
2 lbs. of beef brisket
4 parsnips (sliced)
1 large onion (sliced)
6 fresh thyme sprigs
¾ cup of dry red wine (it is optional)
2 tablespoons of Beau Monde seasoning (see directions below, but it is optional)
¾ cup of fresh parsley (chopped)
Cooking fat

Ingredients for the Beau Monde Seasoning
1 tablespoon of ground cloves
1 teaspoons of ground cinnamon
1 tablespoons of ground bay leaf
1 tablespoons of ground allspice
1 teaspoons of ground nutmeg
1 teaspoon of celery seed
Sea salt and freshly ground black pepper to taste

Directions:

1. First, you combine the entire ingredients for the Beau Monde seasoning in a small bowl.

2. After which you sprinkle beef with salt and pepper to taste.

3. After which you heat some cooking fat over a medium-high heat in a large skillet and brown the beef on each side for about 4 minutes.

4. At this point, you transfer beef to a slow cooker.

5. Then you add the carrot, parsnips, celery, onion, and leek.

6. Furthermore, you mix the beef stock, red wine (if using), tomato puree, garlic, thyme sprigs, parsley, and Beau Monde seasoning in a bowl.

7. After which you pour the mixture over the beef and vegetables.

8. Then you cover and cook on low for about 10 to 12 hours or until tender.

9. Finally, you serve warm with the vegetables.

Bigos Recipe

Ingredients
6 cups of sauerkraut
¾ lb. of bacon sliced
1 ½ lbs. of Kielbasa sausage sliced (it is optionally substitute with a quality sausage from your butcher)
3 cloves garlic (minced)
Salt and pepper to taste (it is optional)
¾ medium cabbage
1 ½-can tomato paste
1 ½ lbs. of pork diced (note that any parts that can be sautéed is good)
1 ½ large onion (diced)
1 ½ bay leaf

Directions:
1. First, you cut your washed cabbage in thin slice and boil until tender in a pot.

2. After which you boil the sauerkraut in another pot in about 3 cups of water.

3. After that, you strain and keep the sour water aside.

4. At this point, you sauté your diced pork in a pan with some cooking oil (lard, coconut oil or butter are good).

5. Then you set aside and sauté the bacon and sausage with the onion and garlic.

6. Furthermore, you combine the cooked cabbage, sauerkraut, sour water, tomato paste, spices and your cooked meats, onion and garlic in a large pot.

7. Finally, you let simmer for about an hour.

Thai Pork Lettuce Wraps Recipe

Ingredients
2 cups of chicken stock
A Fresh lettuce leaves (cut into approximately 3 x 3 inches)
1 tablespoons of fish sauce
4 tablespoons of water
1 lime (quartered)
Sea salt and freshly ground black pepper to taste
1 lb. pork, thinly sliced
¾ lb. of mung bean sprouts
½ cup of almond butter
2 tablespoons of white wine vinegar
1 teaspoon of sambal sauce (it is optional)
1 tablespoon of Paleo cooking fat;

Directions:
1. First, you bring the chicken stock to a boil in a pan placed over a medium-high heat and add the pork slices.

2. After which you simmer and cook for about 5 minutes, until the pork is cooked.

3. After that, you remove the pork pieces and set aside to cool (Note: you will not need the chicken stock anymore, but you can stock it in the refrigerator for later recipes).

4. At this point, you cook the mung bean sprouts with the cooking fat in the same pan, for about 3 to 4 minutes and then set aside.

5. Then you combine the ingredients for the almond butter sauce in a bowl: the almond butter, fish sauce, white wine vinegar, and water and sambal sauce.

6. Season it with sea salt and black pepper to taste.

7. Furthermore, once the cooked ingredients have cooled down, you place some pork; some mung bean sprouts and some almond butter sauce over each lettuce leave and then squeeze some fresh lime juice on top.

8. Finally, you roll them into wraps and enjoy.

Canned salmon salad

Tips: In this recipe, I used olive oil and lemon juice, but homemade mayonnaise are also great. Ingredients

2 diced cucumbers (peeled)

1 large tomato, diced

5-6 tablespoons of extra virgin olive oil

Lettuce leaves for serving

2 cans of wild salmon

1 onion, chopped

1 avocado, diced

2 tablespoons of chopped fresh dill (it is optional)

2 lemons juice

Directions:

1. First, you drain the liquid from the canned salmon.
2. After which you place the salmon in a bowl and mash well with a fork.
3. After that, you add the lemon juice and olive oil and mix well into the salmon.
4. At this point, you add the cucumbers, onion, tomato and avocado and mix again.
5. Finally, you add the dill, if using, and season with salt and pepper.
6. Then you serve the cold salad over lettuce leaves.

White wine & garlic mussels

Ingredients

4 cups of white wine or chicken stock

10 finely chopped cloves garlic

12 tablespoons of butter or ghee

8 lbs. of fresh mussels

4 chopped onions

2/ 3 cup of your favorite chopped fresh herbs (or preferably parsley and basil)

Directions

1. First, you wash, remove the beards and discard any of the opened mussels prior to cooking.
2. After which you combine the whine or stock, onions and garlic in a stockpot, bring to a boil and simmer for about 5 minutes.
3. After that, you add the mussels to the pot cover and increase the heat to medium-high so the sauce boils and creates steam that will cook the mussels.
4. As soon as all the mussels have opened, then you add the butter or ghee and herbs and remove from heat.
5. Finally, you serve in bowls with the white wine, garlic and butter sauce.

Pork chops with apples and onions

Ingredients

6 tablespoons of lard, butter, ghee or coconut oil

Pepper and salt to taste

8 bone-in pork chops (with the trimmings)

8 sliced and cored apples

4 large onion (sliced)

Directions:

1. First, you heat a large pan over a medium-high heat.
2. After which you season the pork chops with salt and pepper to taste.
3. After that, you melt 4 tablespoons of the cooking fat and fry the chops, for about 5 minutes on each side, until well cooked and browned.
4. At this point, you set the pork chops aside, reduce the heat to medium-low, add the other tablespoons of cooking fat and add the onion and apple slices.
5. Then you cook for about 4 minutes, until the onions have caramelized and the apple slices are slightly soft.
6. Finally, you serve the chops with the topping of apple and onions.

Hearty beef stew recipe

Ingredients

4 tablespoons of paleo cooking fat

2 cups of onion (chopped)

6 carrots (peeled and chopped)

2 (28oz) can diced tomatoes

Sea salt and freshly ground black pepper to taste

2 lbs. of stewing beef

8 cups of beef stock

2 cups of celery (chopped)

4 potatoes, peeled and cubed (it is optional)

1 teaspoons of fresh thyme (finely chopped)

1 teaspoons of fresh rosemary (finely chopped)

Directions:

1. First, you combine the onions, celery, carrots, potatoes, in a large saucepan over a medium-high heat if using, as well as the cooking fat.
2. After which you cook for about 3 to 5 minutes, stirring constantly.
3. Then you add the beef to the saucepan, followed by the tomatoes, beef stock, rosemary and thyme.
4. After that, you season to taste with salt and pepper.
5. At this point, you cover the saucepan and cook for an hour, allowing the stew to simmer.
6. Make sure you stir a few times during the cooking process.
7. Finally, you remove the lid and cook uncovered for about 45 minutes and if the mixture is too thick at the end of the cooking process, I suggest you add a little bit of water or stock.

Slow Cooker Beef and Pepper Soup Recipe

Ingredients

2 cups of onion (diced)

2 (15 oz.) diced tomatoes

6 cups of beef stock

1 teaspoon of dried oregano

Sea salt and freshly ground black pepper to taste

2 lbs. of extra-lean ground beef

4 cups of cauliflower (minced)

4 bell peppers, chopped (any color)

2 (15 oz.) of tomato sauce

1 teaspoon of dried basil Cooking fat

6 cloves garlic (crushed)

Directions:

1. First, you melt some cooking fat in a skillet placed over a medium-high heat and cook the onion and the garlic for a minute.
2. After which, you add the beef to the skillet and cook until the meat is browned.
3. After that, you place the beef and onion mixture in a slow cooker.
4. Then you add all the remaining ingredients, season to taste, and give everything a good stir.
5. Finally, you cover and cook on low for about 6 to 8 hours.

Steak with Bell Peppers Skillet Recipe

Ingredients

2 large sweet onions (thinly sliced)

6 bell peppers (sliced)

Sea salt and freshly ground black pepper to taste

2 lbs. flank steak (sliced)

6 shallots (sliced)

2 garlic cloves (minced)

4 tablespoons of cooking fat

Directions:

1. First, you heat up 2 tablespoons of cooking fat in a large skillet placed over a medium heat.
2. After which you toss in the onions and garlic and cook for about 4 to 5 minutes.
3. After that, you transfer the onion and garlic to a plate and set aside.
4. Then you add the other tablespoon of cooking fat in the same skillet and keep at a medium-high heat.
5. At this point, you add the beef to the skillet.
6. After which you cook for about 6 minutes, or until browned to desired doneness, and set aside.
7. Then you add the bell peppers and shallots, and cook until the peppers start to soften (approximately 5 minutes).
8. Finally, you toss the onions and beef back into the pan and cook until everything is warm (approximately 2 minutes), and serve.

Texas-style of Beef Brisket Recipe

Ingredients

2 tablespoons of celery seeds

2 tablespoons of dried oregano

11 to 15 lbs. brisket (untrimmed)

2 tablespoons of coriander seeds (ground)

2 tablespoons of smoked paprika

6 tablespoons of chili powder

2 tablespoons of garlic powder

Sea salt

2 tablespoons of allspice (ground)

2 tablespoons of mustard seeds (ground)

2 cups of beef stock

Freshly ground black pepper (to taste)

Directions:

1. First, you combine the chili powder, mustard seeds, smoked paprika, allspice, coriander, garlic powder, celery seeds, oregano, and season to taste with salt and pepper together.
2. After which you rub the entire brisket with the spice rub and then wrap tightly in plastic wrap.
3. Refrigerate for at least 4 hours or up to 24 h.
4. Meanwhile, you heat your oven to a temperature of 350 F.
5. After which you place the brisket in a roasting pan and roast, uncovered, for about 1 hour.
6. At this point, you add the beef stock to the roasting pan.
7. After that, you cover tightly and lower the heat to a temperature of 300 F.
8. Then you cook for another 2 to 3 hours or until fork tender.
9. Finally, once cooked, you then slice the meat thinly across the grain and serve

Gingered Beef Salad Recipe

Ingredients

2/ 3 cup of ginger vinaigrette salad dressing

8 cups of mixed spring (or baby salad greens)

1 red onion (thinly sliced)

1 lb. of beef sirloin steak (cut into thin strips)

3 cups of broccoli (cut into florets)

1 red bell pepper (thinly sliced)

Ingredients for the Ginger vinaigrette salad dressing

2 tablespoons of shallots, minced

2 tablespoons of lime juice

Sea salt and freshly ground black pepper

1 tablespoon of fresh ginger, minced

1 tablespoon of rice wine vinegar

½ cup of extra -virgin olive oil

Directions:

1. First, you combine all of the ingredients for the vinaigrette in a bowl.
2. After which you season to taste, and whisk well.
3. After that, you warm up 2 tablespoons of the ginger vinaigrette in a skillet placed over a medium high heat.
4. At this point, you add the broccoli to the warm vinaigrette and cook for about 3 minutes.
5. Then you add the beef to the skillet and cook for another 3 minutes, after which you remove the skillet from the heat.
6. This is when you combine the mixed greens, bell pepper, onion, beef and broccoli in a salad bowl.
7. Finally, you drizzle the salad with the remaining vinaigrette, toss, and serve

Beef Chuck with Braised Vegetables Recipe

Ingredients

1 cup of carrots (diced)

1 large onion (diced) Beef chuck (approximately 3 ½ pounds)

1 cup of celery (diced)

2 teaspoons of fresh rosemary (minced)

1 tablespoons of cooking fat

Sea salt and freshly ground black pepper

An Additional ¼ cup Paleo cooking fat or ghee

Directions

1. Meanwhile, you heat your oven to a temperature of 275 F.
2. After which you season the chuck to taste with sea salt and black pepper.
3. After that, you warm the coconut oil on the stovetop, in a Dutch oven over a high heat, and brown the beef on all sides.
4. At this point, you remove the chuck, and add all the remaining ingredients to the Dutch oven and reduce the heat to medium-low.
5. Then you cook the vegetables for about 5 minutes, stirring frequently.
6. This is when you return the beef to the pot.
7. After that, you cover and roast in the oven for about 2 hours or until the beef is, fork tender.
8. Finally, you let the beef rest and serve with the braised vegetables.

Bacon-Wrapped Butternut Squash Recipe

Ingredients

15 slices of bacon (cut in half)

1 teaspoon of garlic powder

Freshly ground black pepper, to taste

2 lbs. of butternut squash (cut into cubes)

1 teaspoons of chili powder

1 teaspoon of paprika

Directions:

1. Meanwhile, you heat your oven to a temperature of 350 F.
2. Place the squash in a bowl and then you sprinkle with garlic powder, chili powder, paprika, and black pepper.
3. After which you wrap bacon slices around the squash cubes and place on a baking sheet.
4. After that, you place in the preheated oven and bake for about 20 minutes.
5. At this point, you flip the bites over and bake for another 20 minutes.
6. Finally, you set the oven to broil for about 2 to 3 minutes if you like your bacon crunchier.

Spicy beef jerky

Ingredients

4 tablespoons of water

½ teaspoon of cayenne pepper

1 teaspoon of freshly ground black pepper

½ cup of Worcestershire sauce

1lb lean top round or sirloin beef roast (fat trimmed and partially frozen)

2 cloves of garlic (finely chopped)

½ teaspoon of sea salt

2 teaspoons of chili powder

Directions:

1. First, with the use of a good knife, cut the roast into thin slices, about 1/ 8 inches thick.
2. After that, you combine the water, garlic, cayenne pepper, sea salt, black pepper, chili powder and Worcestershire sauce in a bowl.
3. Then you add the beef slices to the mixture, cover and refrigerate overnight for the flavors to penetrate then meat.
4. At this point, you place the beef slices, without their marinating liquid, side by side on baking sheets and roast in a 175 F oven for about 3 hours.
5. After which you turn the meat over and roast for another hour or two, until the meat is dry but still bends without breaking.
6. Then you enjoy and place the leftovers in an airtight container in the refrigerator.

Thai Coconut Soup Recipe

Ingredients

1 bunch of scallions (thinly sliced)

4 garlic cloves (minced)

1 large carrot (peeled and shredded)

4 cups of chicken stock

1 tablespoons of fish sauce Fresh minced herbs (such as cilantro or basil)

Sea salt and freshly ground black pepper to taste

1 lb. of boneless skinless chicken breasts

1 red bell pepper (sliced)

2-inch piece of fresh ginger (peeled and finely chopped)

1 jalapeño (seeded and minced)

1 cup of shiitake mushrooms (sliced)

1 can of full-fat coconut milk (14 oz.)

1 teaspoon of lime zest Lime wedges, for serving

2 tablespoons of cooking fat

Directions:

1. First, you heat the cooking fat in a large saucepan over a medium heat.
2. After which you cook the scallions, garlic, and ginger for about 5 minutes, stirring frequently, until softened.
3. After that, you add the carrot, jalapeño, and mushroom, and cook for about 3-4 minutes until softened.
4. Then you add the chicken, chicken stock, coconut milk, and fish sauce.
5. At this point, you bring the soup to a boil then reduce to a simmer and cook for about 15 to 20 minutes until the chicken is cooked through.
6. This is when you remove the chicken from the soup and then shred it into chunks and return to the pot.
7. Then you stir in the lime zest, the fresh herbs, and salt and pepper to taste, and remove from the heat.
8. Finally, you garnish each bowl with a lime wedge to serve.

Chunky Meat and Vegetable Soup Recipe

Ingredients

1 large onion (diced)

3 garlic cloves (minced)

3 cups of beef broth

4 whole carrots (peeled and sliced)

3 tablespoons of tomato paste

Sea salt and freshly ground black pepper to taste

2- ½ lbs. of ground beef

2 celery stalks (diced)

2 sweet potatoes (cut into chunks)

3 bell peppers (seeded and diced)

14.5 ounce can of diced tomatoes (or better still three large tomatoes, diced)

½ teaspoon of ground oregano

1-teaspoon chili powder

Directions:

1. First, you brown the meat with the onion, garlic, and celery in a large saucepan placed over a medium high heat.
2. After which you add the remaining ingredients to the saucepan, season to taste, and stir to combine.
3. Then you bring to a boil, then reduce to a simmer, cover, and cook for about 15 to 20 minutes or until the sweet potatoes are soft.

Creamy Zucchini and Mushroom Soup Recipe

Ingredients

1 large zucchini (chopped)

2 cloves garlic (minced)

2 bay leaves

1 cup of coconut milk

Sea salt and freshly ground black pepper

1 lb. of fresh mushrooms (chopped)

1 medium onion (chopped)

Several sprigs of fresh thyme (or one tablespoon dried thyme)

3 cups of chicken stock (or vegetable stock)

1 tablespoon of ghee

Directions:

1. First, you melt the ghee in a large saucepan, placed over a medium heat and you cook the onion and garlic until softened, about 5 minutes.
2. After which you add the mushrooms, thyme, and bay leaves, and cook for another 5 minutes.
3. After that, you add the zucchini and cook for about10-15 minutes until the vegetables release their juices.
4. Then you add the stock to the saucepan and bring to a boil; then reduce the heat and simmer for 5 minutes.
5. At this point, you remove the thyme sprigs (i.e. if you used them) and bay leaves from the soup.
6. Furthermore, you add the coconut milk and let the soup simmer for another 5 minutes, stirring frequently.
7. Finally, you puree the soup with an immersion blender (or in batches with a regular blender) until smooth.
8. Make sure you serve warm.

Coconut Lime Chicken Soup Recipe

Ingredients

15 oz. (i.e. 1 can + a few tablespoons) of coconut milk

¼ cup of lime juice

1 cup of broccoli (shredded)

2 teaspoons Thai seasoning (detailed below)

Sea salt and freshly ground black pepper

2 lbs. of cooked chicken (cut into pieces)

3 cups of chicken broth

3 medium carrots (shredded)

1 cup of rutabaga (shredded)

1 lime (cut into wedges)

Ingredients for Thai seasoning

¼ teaspoon of cinnamon

¼ teaspoon of chili powder

¼ teaspoon of salt

½ teaspoon of curry powder

¼ teaspoon of ginger

¼ teaspoon of paprika;

Directions:

1. First, you combine the chicken broth, coconut milk, lime juice, Thai seasoning, shredded vegetables and chicken pieces in a large saucepan.
2. After which you season to taste with salt and pepper.
3. At this point, you bring the soup to a boil, then reduce the heat and let it simmer, covered, for about 15 minutes or until the vegetables are getting slightly tender.
4. Make sure you serve warm, with lime wedges.

Bacon-Wrapped Avocado Recipe

Ingredients

Chili powder

8-12 strips of bacon

2 avocados

Directions:

1. Meanwhile, you heat your oven to a temperature of 425 F. After which you line a baking sheet with foil or parchment paper.
2. After that, you cut the avocado into equal slices.
3. Then you wrap each avocado slice with bacon, (1 slice of bacon should be good for 1 or 2 avocado slices.)
4. At this point, you sprinkle some chili powder over the bacon-wrapped slices, and line them up on the baking sheet.
5. Finally, you place in the oven and bake for 12 to 15 minutes.

Ingredients

6-8 slices of good quality prosciutto

1 tablespoons of honey (it is optional)

Sea salt and freshly ground black pepper to taste

3 ripe peaches (halved and pitted)

1 cup of balsamic vinegar

2 tablespoons of coconut oil (or clarified butter, melted)

8-10 basil leaves

Directions:

1. First, you bring the vinegar to a simmer in a small saucepan over a medium-high heat, and let simmer for a few minutes.
2. Once it begins to thicken, you add the honey, if using, and season to taste with salt and pepper.
3. At a point, when the liquid takes on the form of thick syrup, you remove from the heat and allow cooling.
4. After that, you fire up the grill to a medium heat and while you waiting for the grill to heat up, brush some of the coconut oil or clarified butter over the open side of each peach.
5. Then you place them on grill face down and allow cooking until golden brown.
6. After which you cook on the other side for only a minute.
7. Finally, you place the peaches face up on a large flat dish.
8. Then you, drizzle them with the balsamic vinegar syrup and then stuff the area where the pit was with prosciutto.
9. Make sure you top with a basil leave, before you serve.

Avocado Daiquiri

Ingredients:

½ medium-ripe avocado

½ oz. of fresh lemon or lime juice

3 cups of ice cubes

8 oz. of rum (preferably a mix of gold and silver)

1 oz. of half-and-half

4 oz. of simple syrup (an equal part sugar and water)

Directions:

1. First, you combine the entire ingredients and blend until smooth.

Chilled Cucumber-Avocado Soup

Ingredients:

4 avocados

1 1/ 3 Cups of each of yogurt and milk

2 tablespoons of each of lemon juice and chopped mint

Salt and freshly ground pepper

4 unpeeled cucumbers

2 cups of vegetable broth

4 tablespoons of chopped onion

2   teaspoons of vinegar Pinches of cayenne

Directions:

First, you combine 4 unpeeled cucumbers, 4 avocados, 2 cups of vegetable broth, 1 1/ 3 cup each of yogurt and milk, 4 tablespoons of chopped onion, 2 tablespoons of each of lemon juice and chopped mint, 2 teaspoons of vinegar, and a pinch of cayenne in a blender.

2. After which you puree and then season with salt and freshly ground pepper.
3. Finally, you chill at least 4 hours, or even overnight, before enjoying this do-ahead warm-weather treat.

Green Breakfast Burrito

Ingredients:

8 beaten eggs

Salt and pepper

Tomato salsa (or preferably salsa Verde)

3 tablespoons of butter

3 cup of chopped fresh spinach

2 avocados, sliced

Directions:

1. First, you melt the 3 tablespoons of butter in a nonstick skillet on medium heat.
2. After which you stir in 8 beaten eggs and 3 cups of chopped fresh spinach and then add salt and pepper.
3. After that, you cook stirring for about 2 minutes until the eggs are softly scrambled.
4. Than you wrap the eggs in warm corn tortillas.
5. Finally, you top with sliced avocado and tomato salsa or salsa Verde.

Chocolate Avocado Shake

Ingredients:

4 tablespoons of brown sugar

3 cups of skim milk

1 ripe Hass avocado

4 tablespoons of coca powder

2 teaspoons of vanilla extract

Directions:

1. First, you place all ingredients in a blender and blend until smooth.
2. Make sure you serve over ice

Tomato and Avocado Sashimi Salad

Ingredients:

2 avocadoes (thinly sliced)

4 tablespoons of fresh cilantro leaves

3 lbs. tomatoes (thinly sliced)

2 tablespoons of fresh lime juice

2 tablespoons of extra virgin olive oil

Directions:

1. First, you layer tomatoes and avocado on platter.
2. After which you drizzle lime juice and oil over top.
3. Then you sprinkle with cilantro and salt to taste.

Egg, Avocado, and Spicy Mayo Sandwich

Ingredients:

2 teaspoons of mayonnaise

2 avocadoes Pinch of cayenne pepper

2 whole-wheat English muffin

2 eggs

Directions:

1. First, you mix a pinch of cayenne pepper into 2 teaspoons of mayonnaise.
2. After which you split and toast a whole-wheat English muffin, and then spread each piece with the spicy mayo.
3. After that, you fry an egg until the yolk is still a little bit runny and place it on a muffin half.
4. Then you top with a few slices of avocado and close the sandwich.

Carrot Soufflé

Ingredients:

2/ 3 cup of honey

6 tablespoons of flour

2 teaspoons of baking powder

6 large eggs (lightly beaten)

14 cups of chopped carrots (about 4 lbs.)

½ cup of sour cream

4 tablespoons of coconut oil

2 teaspoons of vanilla extract

½ teaspoon of salt

Directions:

1. First, you heat oven to a temperature of 350 °F.
2. After which you Oil/ butter a 2-quart baking dish.
3. After that, you cook carrots in boiling water for about 10-15 minutes until very tender; drain.
4. At this point, you place cooked carrots in food processor (be careful, carrots will be hot) and process until smooth.

Note that you can also use a potato ricer.

5. Then you add remaining ingredients and process until mixed.
6. This is when you spoon into prepared pan.
7. Finally, you bake for about 40 minutes, making sure soufflé is puffed and set.

Cheesy Fried Rice

Ingredients:

8 tablespoons of coconut oil

Salt

4 eggs

4 cups of cooked brown rice (leftover works great!)

8 oz. shredded extra sharp cheddar cheese

Directions:

1. First, you whisk eggs together in small bowl and then set aside.
2. After which you melt coconut oil in medium sauté pan.
3. Then once the oil is hot, you add rice and stir-fry the rice.
4. At this point, you move all rice to edges of pan and pour beaten eggs in the middle.
5. In addition, you scramble eggs and when they are almost done re-incorporate rice.
6. After which you add cheese and stir until all melted.
7. Finally, you sprinkle with salt to taste.

Chicken Nuggets fried in Coconut Oil

Ingredients:

2 teaspoons of crushed red pepper flakes

4 eggs

4 lbs. ground chicken

4 teaspoons of chili powder

2 cups of breadcrumbs (or preferably ground up brown rice cereal)

Fresh ground pepper

2 teaspoons of salt Coconut oil, as required

1 teaspoon of onion powder

1 teaspoon of garlic powder

Directions:

1. First, you mix all ingredients except coconut oil together until well blended.
2. After which, you add more breadcrumbs if mixture looks too sticky.
3. After that, you heat coconut oil in a pan over medium heat and drop chicken mixture into pan, shaping into nuggets.
4. Then you cook until golden brown on both sides and serve.

Chili-Coconut Crusted Shrimp

Tips: This recipe is a terrific appetizer; it can be served with a bowl of rice and stir-fried vegetables as a main course.

Ingredients:

¼ cup of dried Thai Chilies

½ cup of flour

1 egg

2-3 tablespoons of coconut oil

24 large shrimp (or preferably prawns)

1 cup of unsweetened finely shredded coconut

Salt to taste

Water

Directions:

1. First, you peel the shrimp, leaving the tails on.
2. After which, you rinse and pat dry and then place chilies in a spice grinder and grind into a fine powder.
3. After that, you use a shallow bowl to mix shredded coconut, flour, salt, and 2 tablespoons of the chili powder.
4. Then you heat oil in a large skillet.
5. At this point, you whisk the egg in a bowl with a little bit of water.
6. In addition, you dip each shrimp in the egg mixture and coat it lightly with the chili-coconut mixture.
7. Finally, you fry for about two minutes on one side and another minute on the other side, or until golden brown and crispy.

Chocolate Almond Granola

Ingredients:

4 tablespoons of coconut oil (melted)

2 teaspoon of vanilla extract

2 tablespoon of cocoa powder

½ cup of chocolate chips

10 tablespoons of brown rice syrup

2 tablespoons of almond butter

3 cups of oats

½ cup of almonds (chopped)

Directions:

1. Meanwhile, you heat oven to a temperature of 325 degrees F.
2. After which you combine the brown rice syrup, oil, almond butter and vanilla in a large bowl until well mixed.
3. After that, you fold in the oats and add the rest of the ingredients stirring to coat.
4. Once mixture is well-combined, then you pour onto a lined baking sheet.
5. Bake for about 22 minutes in preheated oven, stirring once.
6. Finally, you let cooing before you serve.

Roasted Red Kurri Coconut Curry Soup

Ingredients:

3 ¼ teaspoons of garam masala

6 cloves garlic

A hot chili pepper (diced, it is optional)

One teaspoon of roasted cumin

4 shallots (minced)

Salt

½ cup of fresh cilantro, chopped

2 teaspoons of coconut oil (or preferably olive oil)

One medium onion (minced)

8 cups of fat free, low sodium vegetable (or preferably chicken broth)

9 lbs. kuris red squash (or preferably 4)

4 ½ teaspoons of madras curry powder

2 cups of light coconut milk Fresh pepper to taste

Directions:

1. First, you heat the oven to a temperature of 400 ° F.
2. After which you use a heavy, sharp knife to cut the squash into quarters.
3. After that, you place it on a baking sheet and bake for about an hour.
4. At a point, when the squash is cooked and cool enough to handle, then you peel the skin away from the squash flesh (about 6 cups).
5. Then you add oil to a medium soup pot, on medium heat.
6. In addition, when the oil is hot enough, you add onion, shallots, chili pepper and garlic.
7. After which you sauté on low heat until golden and then you add roasted cumin, masala and madras curry powder.
8. After that, you mix thoroughly and cook for another minute.
9. This is when you add broth, roasted Kurri pumpkin, light coconut milk, and cook covered for about 21 - 25 minutes.

10. Then you remove cover and use an immersion blender, puree soup until smooth.
11. Finally, you season with salt and fresh pepper to taste.
12. Make sure you serve with fresh cilantro.

Mango Coconut Chia Pudding

Ingredients:

1 cup of unsweetened almond milk

4 tablespoons of chia seeds

8-12 drops of Nu-Naturals liquid stevia (or preferably sugar/ honey to taste)

1 cup of lite coconut milk

1 ¼ cup of fresh ripe champagne mango (diced)

2 tablespoons of sweetened shredded coconut

Directions:

1. First, you combine the entire ingredients in a large container.
2. After which you mix well and close the container.
3. Then you refrigerate overnight or at least 5-6 hours.
4. Finally, you divide into 2 bowls or glass dishes and serve.

Better Bacon-Egg-and-Cheese Sandwich

Ingredients:

Two slices of whole-wheat bread (toasted)

Salt and pepper to taste

1 tablespoon of fresh goat cheese

Two slices of Canadian bacon

One large egg plus 1 large egg white (lightly beaten)

½ medium tomatoes (sliced)

Directions:

1. First, you cook bacon for about 2 minutes in a medium nonstick skillet and over medium heat until warmed through.
2. After which you transfer bacon to one slice toast.
3. After that, you season eggs with salt and pepper, and then you add to skillet and cook for about 2 minutes until set around edge.
4. At this point, you flip and cook for about 30 seconds.
5. Then you fold into quarters and place on bacon, and then you top with tomato and season with salt and pepper.
6. Finally, you spread goat cheese on remaining toast, and sandwich.

CONCLUSION

Thanks for reading through this book; if you follow judiciously to the recipes outlined above, you will sleep better, feel better, think better, have more energy and loss weight without effort.

Remember, the only bad action you can take is no action at all.

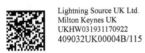

Lightning Source UK Ltd.
Milton Keynes UK
UKHW031931170922
409032UK00004B/115